ORPHAN DISEASES

ORPHAN DISEASES
NEW HOPE FOR
RARE MEDICAL CONDITIONS

WENDY MURPHY

Twenty-First Century Medical Library
Twenty-First Century Books
Brookfield, Connecticut

T 47253

Library of Congress Cataloging-in-Publication Data
Murphy, Wendy B.
Orphan diseases : new hope for rare medical conditions /
Wendy Murphy.
p. cm.
Includes bibliographical references and index.
Summary: Looks at rare diseases, such as Tay-Sachs, cystic fibrosis, and
sickle-cell disease, which are neglected by researchers and drug
manufacturers for fiscal, political, and practical reasons.
ISBN 0-7613-1919-0
1. Rare diseases—Juvenile literature. 2. Orphan drugs—Juvenile
literature. [1. Rare diseases. 2. Diseases. 3. Medicine—Research.]
I. Title.
RC48.8 .M87 2002 362.1'9—dc21 2001007157

Cover photograph courtesy of Photodisc
Photographs courtesy of AP/Wide World Photos: pp. 14, 70, 75, 112; © Lowell
Handler: p. 20; Photofest: p. 37; © Rosalie Winard: p. 42; © Al Lamme/
Phototake: p. 51; Brown Brothers: p. 62; Photo Researchers, Inc./SPL: pp. 83
(© Hattie Young), 107 (© Will & Deni McIntyre), 123 (© Andrew Leonard)

Published by Twenty-First Century Books
A Division of The Millbrook Press, Inc.
2 Old New Milford Road
Brookfield, Connecticut 06804
www.millbrookpress.com

CONTENTS

ORPHAN DISEASES

APART FROM
THE BEATEN PATH

Nature is nowhere accustomed more openly to display her mysteries than in cases where she shows traces of her workings apart from the beaten path; nor is there any better way to advance the proper practice of medicine than to give our minds to the discovery of the usual laws of nature by careful investigation of cases of rarer forms of diseases. For it has been found in almost all things that what they contain of useful or applicable nature is hardly perceived unless we are deprived of them, or they become deranged in some way.
      —William Harvey, London 1657[1]

Rare diseases, though they affect relatively few people, can teach us a lot. As the great English physician William Harvey wrote nearly four centuries ago, these conditions, by their very oddity, can reveal unique information that leads ultimately to scientific discoveries of use not only to those who have the disorder but to a far larger audience. But in being rare, in being off the beaten path, conditions like Huntington's Disease, muscular dystrophy, hemophilia, porphyria, and some hundreds of other disorders have tended to be overlooked by the very people and organizations who are best equipped to study them. The reasons are many.

First, medical research of any kind is enormously expensive. The cost in terms of time and dollars to gather sufficient data; to staff laboratories with skilled and dedicated researchers; and to develop the diagnostic tests, drugs, and other forms of therapy that offer promise of relief can be astronomical. This is a bearable expense when huge rewards lie at the end. Imagine the profits possible for developing a drug that "cures" diabetes, for example. With millions of new diabetics diagnosed each year, the market for any new wonder drug is enormous; and this is borne out in the wealth of research activity that surrounds diabetes. But the same kinds of costs are typically involved in bringing to market a drug for a rare disease, while the financial rewards cannot come close to matching them. Often, the drug company must take its "rewards" in knowing it has performed a humanitarian service.

Then there is the matter of finding test subjects on which to conduct the necessary clinical trials to prove value in the new discovery. For some disorders, there may be only a few hundred persons alive whose cases could be examined for clues, and they may very well be scattered across the country and the globe. How does a researcher with limited time and money gather enough firsthand data to know for sure whether he is dealing with a single disease or several diseases whose symptoms just happen to bear some similarities to each other?

Another factor that works against rare diseases might be called the squeaky-wheel factor. When funds and time are limited resources, it's only natural that those constituencies that are the most vocal, that have the most "clout," tend to get the most attention. It is no coincidence, for example, that year after year, heart disease gets a large part of the medical research grants given out by the federal government: The senators and congressmen who heartily support these allocations are by dint of their age, sex, and lifestyles prime candidates for heart disease and they know it. So, too, huge amounts of money are raised publicly and privately for cancer research and the development of cancer drugs because virtually everyone in America is in some way touched by cancer.

Lastly, it has become increasingly apparent that most rare diseases have a genetic component in their existence. And until very recently, it has been virtually impossible to decipher what those components might be or how they play into the expression of these disorders. Thus there has been a certain inevitability to most rare diseases—people are born with them and, like the color of their eyes, there has seemed to be little if anything anyone could do about them, practically or ethically.

Now, happily, circumstances are changing. Rare, or "orphan" disorders are finally gaining a place at the research table. Families and individuals who live with these conditions are speaking out and being heard, as never before. Taking as their models organizations like the American Heart Association and the American Cancer Society, they are banding together to lobby for more research funds, and they are networking with each other globally via the Internet to share information about their disorders and to find mutual support.

The federal government has also become involved in promoting research, both by providing specific funding and through other kinds of incentives that encourage pharmaceutical companies to develop "orphan drugs." With the mapping of the genome now well under way, the specific genetic sites at which some rare disorders originate are also becoming clear. And substantial strides are even being made in gene therapy, giving rise to the hope that the day when genetic errors can be deleted and corrections inserted may be close at hand.

In the pages that follow, we will take a look at a few of the six thousand or so rare diseases that are currently recognized as distinct conditions by the National Institutes of Health (NIH) and describe what is known about them, how they are being treated today, and what their long-term prospects are. It's an exciting story, to say the least.

Chapter One

OPTIMISM IN MOTHER TERESA'S WAITING ROOM

NEW HOPE FOR ORPHAN DISORDERS

We're sitting in Room 2358 of the Rayburn House Office Building in Washington, DC. It's Friday, April 13, 2001, and the room is crowded. Subcommittee members and their staff are clustered around a bank of raised tables on one side of the room. Dozens of individuals representing various organizations and "causes" are seated opposite; a few of the visitors are in wheelchairs, a few disabled in other ways; two appear to be parents of a young child whom they are holding in their arms. The child seems abnormally pale and listless. Assorted doctors and lawyers and scientists are also in the audience. Each of them has come to speak on behalf of a particular medical disorder and to advocate passionately for more funding. When one of them is invited up to the microphone, he or she talks fast because these advocates are given only five minutes to make their case. Over this long day, dozens of advo-

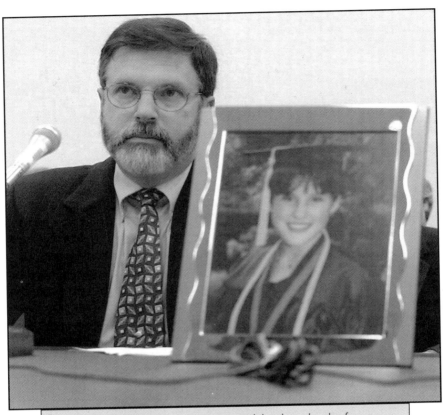

The father of a seventeen-year-old who died of a rare form of cancer testifies before a House appropriations subcommittee on Capital Hill, asking for increased NIH funding for research.

cates are heard as the congressmen listen intently, interrupting occasionally, taking frequent notes.[1]

Though the sign on the door identifies the event as "Public Witness Testimony before the House Appropriations Subcommittee on Labor, Health and

Human Services and Education," the familiar name for what is going on is "Mother Teresa's Waiting Room." Such is the heartbreaking testimony of suffering, courage, and hope presented here for five days each spring, and such are the life-and-death decisions that the appropriations subcommittee members must finally make as they decide how to divide up the year's budget of several million dollars for medical research among literally thousands of worthy enterprises.

As awkward as the process seems, Mother Teresa's Waiting Room represents an enormous advance over what had gone before. Before the 1980s, rare diseases went virtually unnoticed except among the relatively small population of individuals and their families who were directly affected. When a baby was born with one of these conditions, or when a seemingly healthy youngster began to fail for reasons that lay outside the family physician's experience and expertise, there was rarely an expert to turn to, or a medical center that could hold out hope of diagnosis and treatment. The causes were essentially deemed a mystery, and parents were left to deal with the problem on their own.

Many rare disorders lacked even something as basic as an identifying name, and if there were scientists focused on finding causes or cures, they usually worked in isolation and with little or no funding unless they happened to have a wealthy patron with a personal interest in finding answers. Drug researchers had, if possible, even less financial support. It simply was not cost effective for pharmaceutical companies to spend millions of dollars developing treatments that would be used by, at best, only a few thousand patients. As for the federal government and its powerful NIH, so long as their budgets were small, the needs of the majority came first. Infectious diseases, heart and cardiovascular health, arthritis, cancer, diabetes, various common bone disorders, the diseases of aging—all had huge constituencies and obvious needs.

Then in 1980 this bleak situation began to change, thanks to the fortuitous collaboration of a congressman, a concerned mother, and a famous TV actor.[2] It all started when California Representative Henry Waxman, an active member of the Commerce Subcommittee on Health, was approached by a woman named Abbey Meyers. Meyers said she needed help obtaining a drug that was experimental in the United States but was on the market in Canada. Her son suffered from the rare disorder Tourette syndrome (TS). Because of TS, the youngster's body was uncontrollably given to involuntary jerking motions; his face twitched with motor tics and grimaces; and he made compulsive grunting and yipping sounds that were distracting to others, not to say embarrassing to him. He could not live a normal life by any stretch of the imagination.

A drug called pimozide was the only medicine known to relieve the boy's symptoms, but the multinational pharmaceutical company that had introduced it experimentally, had found that the drug was not effective for a prevalent disease, and the cost of winning approval from the Food and Drug Administration (FDA) to market it in the United States for TS was just too expensive to justify the effort. Pimozide continued to be available in Canada, where the rules were more lenient, but when Meyers and other TS parents tried to import it, the drugs were seized by U.S. customs as illegal. Meyers told Waxman that she was sympathetic with the manufacturer's need to protect its stockholders' interests, and she also understood the FDA's need to require extensive clinical testing for safety's sake, but she could not sit idly by as her son and others like him suffered. She wanted Waxman's help in coming up with a solution that could serve all these disparate interests.

Waxman became interested. He held Congressional hearings to find out if groups other than those connected with TS were similarly discriminated against by pharmaceutical companies. Many patient and parent organizations turned up at the hearings to tell stories similar to Meyers's. The hearings were naturally covered in the newspapers, and one reader who took notice was the brother of TV actor Jack Klugman. Klugman thought that the problems of this underserved population would make an interesting and provocative theme for his popular medical drama series, *Quincy*. He commissioned his writers to investigate the topic and to create a dramatic episode based on what they learned. When the resulting show aired in March 1981, thousands of viewers were provoked by the story to send in letters urging that the laws be changed.

With lack of access to therapeutic drugs now a well-publicized issue, Waxman thought the time was ripe to rally industry leaders, medical researchers, patients, and government agencies around a permanent legislative solution. Early in 1982 a bill offering incentives to entice drug companies to increase their research in the area of rare diseases was drafted, but the law was stalled in Congress because of intense opposition by the pharmaceutical industry. Klugman, who by now felt a personal stake in winning its approval, went to Capitol Hill to testify about the need for orphan drug legislation. At the Congressional hearing, several hundred real victims of rare disorders were recruited through their respective support groups to assist. And in a second *Quincy* episode filmed subsequently, some five hundred patients and family members played themselves in a public demonstration on behalf of the bill. It was enough to capture the news a second time and to put the real bill back on track. On January 4, 1983, President Ronald Reagan reluctantly signed the bill into law. Though he had planned to veto it, the publicity changed his mind.

Called the Orphan Drug Act, this important legislation defines an "orphan disease" as any condition that is sufficiently rare that fewer than 200,000 individuals within the U.S. population are affected at any one time.[3] Consequently, neither drug companies nor university or hospital research centers are likely to focus costly research and development efforts on them without some outside incentives. All told, six thousand disorders are known to meet the criteria. The incentives that have been put into place to encourage pharmaceutical companies to become interested in them include substantial tax breaks and rights to market resulting drugs exclusively for seven years in the United States. Even before the act was finalized, the FDA created a special Office of Orphan Products Development to propel research and development of orphan drugs, medical devices, and supplements for rare disorders. And lastly, the act mandates that Congress appropriate funds to conduct research into rare diseases under the FDA Orphan Drug Grant Program.

The incentives have worked better than anyone had dared to hope. Since the bill was signed in 1983, 218 orphan products, including drugs and biologics, have been approved for specific orphan disorders, and more than 400 research grants have been approved by the FDA's Office of Orphan Products Development. (Prior to the act, only ten orphan drugs had been approved and no research grants had been specifically earmarked for work in rare disorders.) More than a thousand other drugs and products are currently going through various stages of research, and while some will almost certainly fail to win final approval, it is equally certain that some of these drugs will bring life-altering relief to people.

Remarkably, a few of the orphan drugs developed under this program have turned out to be very profitable "blockbusters," though this was never the expectation. The genetically engineered hormone erythropoetin was initially developed by Amgen for kidney patients on hemodialysis, but once it was in the market, its larger application as an antianemia drug led to huge sales. And AZT, which is perhaps the most important drug in the arsenal of therapeutic treatments for AIDS, was developed under orphan drug incentives back when the population who could benefit from it was thought to be of very limited scope.

Meanwhile, the parent who had first approached Congressman Waxman, Abbey Meyers, did not rest with the enactment of the Orphan Drug Act. She had learned, in the process of drawing attention to the plight of her son, that there was untapped strength in numbers. Though there were perhaps only 100,000 people with her son's diagnosis in all of America, when all the orphan-disease sufferers were added up, they and their families constituted a lobbying force 25 million strong. Meyers and other veterans of the orphan disease wars used their new momentum to form the National Organization for Rare Disorders (NORD), which was founded in 1983.

Today, NORD is a unique alliance of approximately 140 nonprofit voluntary health organizations and individuals.[4] Under its auspices individuals and physicians can obtain basic, easy to understand, expert descriptions and references for over eleven hundred rare disorders. Starting with epidermolysis bullosa (#1), Tourette syndrome (#2), neurofibromatosis (#3), Parkinson's disease (#4), and autism (#5), it covers a wide range of conditions from such oddly named disorders as Cri du

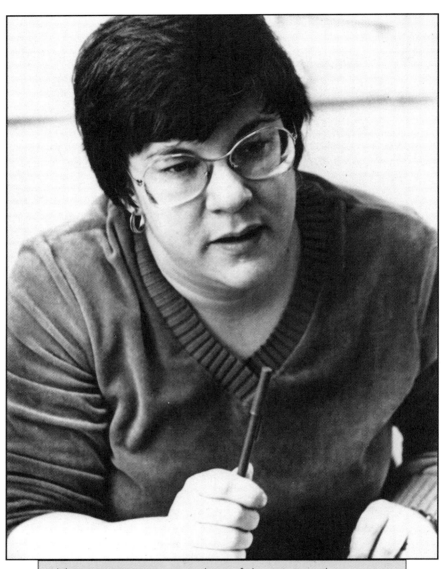

Abbey S. Meyers, president of the National Organization for Rare Disorders (NORD)

Chat syndrome (#19) and Jumping Frenchmen of Maine (#380) to adrenoleukodystrophy (#43), dramatized in the film *Lorenzo's Oil*, true hermaphrodism (#772), Marcus Gunn phenomenon (#833), and Schindler disease (#1028), this last a devastating neurological disorder.

NORD also maintains a unique patient/family networking program that links people with the same rare disease for mutual support, and it undertakes patient advocacy at the national level. At the same time, NORD administers patient assistance programs for pharmaceutical and biotech companies; these are programs of last resort and are designed to assist individuals who cannot afford the often extraordinary costs of prescribed medications.

Lastly, NORD plays an important part in bringing together limited numbers of patients who wish to participate in clinical trials and drug developers who are testing new treatments. In this way potentially important new orphan drugs are able to come to market sooner and at less cost for all concerned. Though NORD's primary focus is the United States, the alliance has naturally taken a leading role in the formation of similar legislation in Europe, Japan, and Australia, countries that modeled their orphan drug laws on the American original.

While the 1983 act will always be regarded as the turning point in rare diseases, NORD is justly proud of its supportive role in lobbying for creation of the Office for Rare Diseases at the NIH, the nation's preeminent center of federally funded medical research. Up until the office's establishment in 1995, there was little if any coordination between the dozen or more separate institutes within the NIH in regard to investigation of rare disorders that often involve several body systems. Thus, researchers at the National Institute of Neurological Disorders (NINDS) might unknowingly have duplicated studies in aspects of autism that were also being studied by researchers at the National Institute of Mental Health (NIMH) or the National Institute of Deafness and Other Communication Disorders (NIDCD).

Even more regrettably, researchers in all these groups might have each decided to take a "hands off" approach toward a particular rare disorder on the grounds that it falls within the territory of some other institute; the result was that no group carried investigations forward. Now, with the help of the Office for Rare Diseases, such studies often benefit from the combined work of many different disciplines sharing many unique perspectives. Also of critical importance, the FDA's Office of Orphan Products Development funds up to $12 million annually for clinical trials at universities and small drug or device development companies. (In many cases, a remedial drug can be devised only after the fundamental cause of the disorder has been located, a process which can take many years.)

CAUSE AND EFFECT

With the marked increase in research funding and investigative activities, a great deal of important new information that applies to most rare disorders has come to light. Most importantly, we can now confirm that most rare diseases are of genetic origin. They are genetic because they are ultimately traceable to the pairs of genes found in the nucleus of each cell. Genes, which are the functional units of the molecule deoxyribonucleic acid or DNA, are strung by the hundreds and even thousands along the twenty-three pairs (or forty-six) chromosomes in the nucleus of each cell in the body. Altogether they make up the genome, or complete code of genetic inheritance. Each gene codes for a particular *trait*, as we refer to some of the more obvious physical characteristics of genetic inheritance like eye color or stature or blood type; but at a molecular level, what genes really code for are the underlying proteins that produce those traits.

One class of proteins is "structural," meaning that it forms such physical structures within the body as bones, muscle, blood vessels, hair, and skin. Another class of proteins is the enzymes, which control an almost infinite number of separate chemical reactions. Enzymes variously keep the heart pumping blood; release energy from food through digestion; make movement and growth possible; control the sending and receiving of chemical messages between cells; fight infections; and operate the senses of sight, hearing, taste, smell, and sound, to name just the most important tasks they perform. The instructions for making proteins are written with a four-letter "alphabet"—scientists use the letters *A*, *G*, *C*, and *T* as shorthand for the four chemical bases adenine, guanine, cytosine, and thymine that go to make DNA.

Every now and then a tiny variation can occur in the making of a gene. Most commonly the variation is a single letter difference, or "snip"—genetics slang for "single nucleotide polymorphism"—that is either added or deleted from the normal sequence of instructions at the time of conception. If the error is in a particularly critical location and produces a notably destructive change in body chemistry, the fetus will die early in the gestation process, dooming the mutation to extinction with it. But if the genetic alteration represents only a small deviation, it may survive to be passed on to the next generation—as a new trait or sometimes as a genetic disease. Snips of this sort are responsible for an estimated five thousand hereditary diseases, including a good share of the orphan diseases with which this book is concerned. (Though a hereditary disease would hardly seem to be "useful," we will learn later that geneticists sometimes discover that the mutation in question protects the individual from some other condition, which, in the ancient time and place in which it was created, had some evolutionary advantage.

Sickle cell anemia, for example, which is discussed in detail in Chapter 3, is one such disorder.) With more extensive research, still other relatively more common diseases, including many cancers, may also turn out to have genetic "misspellings" as a causative factor. The difference in these latter cases is that the mutation becomes a factor only later in life when the individual carrier chances to interact with some environmental circumstance such as prolonged exposure to a toxic chemical in the air, water, or food. The interaction effectively triggers the mutation to go to work in some destructive way, or in some instances causes a belated mutation.

Organisms, including humans, inherit pairs of each gene, one from the mother and one from the father. Often, one of the genes is dominant and the other is recessive, with the result that the dominant gene's instructions will be expressed in the offspring while the recessive instructions are switched off. Sometimes, however, the two genes will be of equal effect with results that are a blend of the two sets of instructions, different to some degree from either parent.

Though it was often possible to deduce from family history that a particular disease was probably the result of inheritance, isolating the specific gene responsible was not possible until recently. As late as 1989, geneticists had managed to link only four genes with their particular diseases. One of them was the single gene for cystic fibrosis (see Chapter 5), and it had taken them nine years to find it. Huntington's disease, which expresses itself only in adulthood, was another of the early discoveries. By 1998 the number of genes that could be linked to specific disorders had grown to one hundred, still only a tiny fraction of the diseases for which information was needed, but the time it took to isolate and decipher their significance once the search was started was growing shorter.

Meanwhile, the development of computational biology—a marriage between computers and molecular biology—was making the collection and interpretation of data much easier. Likewise, the database essential to mapping the entire collection of human genes was growing. The more scientists learned, the better they became at predicting where the next "candidate gene" might be; what had been little better than a guessing game began to be a rational pursuit. Geneticists could look more closely at, say, a few hundred genes instead of thousands to locate the telltale errors.

That genetic research has made such enormous strides in the last fifteen years is thanks chiefly to the Human Genome Project (HGP). The HGP, which was formed as a collaborative effort by the NIH, set itself the audacious goal of using technology to decipher the entire "book of life." Contrary to early predictions, the task that some thought would take many decades and possibly never succeed, was essentially completed early in 2001. The importance of this accomplishment cannot be exaggerated. It has changed the future of medicine forever. With a detailed catalog of the entire range of human genes in hand, researchers have quickly gone from studying conditions caused by mutations in single genes to studying the genetic interactions involved in the most complex diseases.

As important as the HGP is to the future of research into rare diseases, certain general facts about the mechanics of heredity in producing some rare diseases have been known for some time. Based on deductions made back in 1865 by Gregor Mendel, an Augustinian monk and amateur botanist, traits including heritable disorders are passed on with mathematical predictability. Where the causative agent is a dominant gene, say for some essential enzyme, geneticists can presume that the disorder is inherited directly from a parent who has the abnormal gene and thus also has the disease. But children can also inherit a genetic disorder from seemingly healthy parents. In this case, both parents are actually "carriers" of the same mutant gene; the gene is expressed in an offspring only when he or she happens to receive two of them, though another sibling might be fortunate enough to receive the healthy recessive half of each parent's genetic pair.

GENE-BASED MEDICINE

As scientists become better at discovering the genetic underpinnings of many rare diseases, diagnosis, treatment, and even cure are likely to become increasingly possible. Already, it is possible to screen for some rare metabolic diseases early enough in life to correct certain deficiencies and reduce their impact on an individual's life. Several states now routinely use a procedure known as tandem mass spectrometry to scan a drop of blood drawn from the heel of newborns. This automated test, which is now given to over four million babies a year, can detect some thirty inherited disorders, including phenylketonuria (PKU), an enzyme deficiency disorder that can cause mental retardation; hypothyroidism, which can stunt growth and brain development; and medium chain Acyl-CoA dehydrogenase deficiency (MCADD), a metabolic disease that is sometimes the cause of sudden infant death syndrome (SIDS) and which can also lead to mental retardation and massive seizures. That all states have not adopted mass spectrometry as an essential part of their public health programs is, in part, a measure of the relative costliness of testing all newborns. On the other hand, when one considers that among the relatively small population currently tested each year, roughly one thousand newborns are found to have a serious disorder, the cost would seem to be worth every penny. By informing parents and their pediatricians early, and beginning the most effective treatments at once, the larger human and financial costs of caring for severely disabled children and adults is reduced considerably. And sometimes, early diagnosis can actually make it possible to treat and reverse a condition that would otherwise lead to lifelong disability in a youngster.

Gene-based medicine also holds out the hope of someday developing drugs that are guided by a better understanding of how genes work and what exactly happens at the molecular level to cause disease. This approach falls within the specialty science known as pharmacogenomics. While much excitement has focused in recent years on trying to replace faulty genes—of which much more is discussed in Chapter 7—it may well turn out that a simpler therapeutic solution will be to create a drug that replaces the protein the normal gene would have produced had it worked properly. Alternatively, it may be possible to produce a drug that somehow interacts with the faulty protein to change its behavior for the better. Not only will such "rational" drugs be able to correct the disorder in part or in full, but in being so finely targeted, they are less likely to cause the side effects that usually go with strong medicine.

With this brief explanation of what rare disorders are and how scientists are working to diagnose and treat them, we will now move on to look at several orphan disorders in detail.

Chapter Two

THE RAIN MAN SYNDROME

AUTISM AND OTHER NEURODEVELOPMENTAL DISORDERS

I live in a home within myself. Each time I begin to write, my brain becomes filled with images. I think visually—my emotions show color and texture against my mind's eye like a projector. Mine is a world of senses and feelings. It is rich with private perceptions. . . . I spoke as a child, and then stopped when I could no longer stand the unbelievable anxiety . . . that came with the effort of talking. . . . I remain within my inner world at all times, like living inside a lovely seashell. I'm an alien who peers out at another world with shy, introverted eyes.

— Jasmine Lee O'Neill,
a young Englishwoman,
describes her experience
living with classic autism.[1]

The word *autism* translates loosely as "withdrawal into self," and in its broadest definition it describes a complex developmental disability that is the result of a neurological disorder affecting the brain. The resulting disability ranges from severe to mild, with the most severe effects being associated with low intelligence and general helplessness and the mildest forms resembling nothing more than a learning disability in an otherwise "normal" person.

America's Centers for Disease Control and Prevention (CDC), the federal agency that tracks health statistics, has estimated that the condition occurs in as many as one in five hundred individuals and is four times more prevalent in boys than in girls. The CDC also notes that autism is on the rise. That's partly because it is being correctly identified more often, but changing environmental factors may also play a part. Up to 100,000 children 18 and under are now estimated to be affected in the United States, a figure that is double the number cited only a couple of decades ago.

Like Jasmine, most people with autism have extremely limited activities and interests. Their social behavior is often unconventional. When it comes to interpreting what others mean by their actions, expressions, or tone of voice, they haven't a clue. They can seem thoughtless, ill-mannered, insensitive, and alien because of their differentness. In sum, living with them can be a constant challenge, as their parents and siblings know only too well, but theirs is a biological condition over which they have very little control. Traditionally, the long-term outlook for those with severe autism has been eventual institutionalization, because there are no known "cures." However, as medical research increases our understanding of autism, it is becoming increasingly possible to treat some of the symptoms and behaviors so that higher-functioning autistic people can find their place in a more accepting world.

When child psychologists and pediatricians first began to identify autism as a unique condition back in the 1930s and 1940s, they theorized that the cause was some kind of "psychogenic" injury that occurred after birth. Many of the children studied came from highly successful, socially advantaged families, so much so that doctors began to suspect there was a link between the parents' busy lives and their children's autism. Perhaps the parents were too self-engrossed to spend the time and attention on parenting that their children needed for normal development. So-called "refrigerator moms" were specifically singled out for what psychologists described as their cool detachment and lack of caring. But we now know that these families were not statistically more likely to produce autistic children. It was just that parents with more secure financial circumstances and better educations were more likely to seek medical advice for their children's difficult behaviors in those days. The less advantaged families tended to suffer in silence, presuming there was nothing to be done about their severely withdrawn children.

DEFINING AUTISM

Psychologists Dr. Leo Kanner of Johns Hopkins Hospital in Baltimore, Maryland, and Dr. Hans Asperger of Vienna, Austria, were the first to identify the set of behavioral characteristics that we now recognize as shared to a greater or lesser degree by all autistic people. Though Drs. Kanner and Asperger worked independently in different parts of the world, they were in almost perfect agreement on their descriptions of the autistic syndrome. (When a disorder has multiple symptoms occurring together, it is often referred to as a "syndrome." When the degree of disability varies greatly from mild to severe, the range is referred to as a "spectrum.") Kanner's description is particularly apt, for he broke the syndrome into three distinct parts: "autistic aloneness," "a desire for sameness," and "islands of ability." All or most of these symptoms are apparent before the third birthday and persist throughout life, though some aspects can be modified if the individual receives knowledgeable support and therapy as he or she matures.

By *autistic aloneness*, Dr. Kanner meant "an inability to relate . . . in the ordinary way to people and situations from the beginning of life."[2] Kanner observed that the child with autism disregards, ignores, and willfully shuts out anything that tries to penetrate the fortress he has erected against physical or emotional sensations.

Though it is usually not possible to identify with certainty all the criteria for autism before the age of three, parents and doctors often report that they noticed "things were not quite right" at an earlier stage. They recall that the infant resisted cuddling, often arching his back and becoming rigid when picked up; he turned away from eye contact, too, which is in contrast to babies' more typical behavior of gazing intently on caregivers and mimicking facial expressions. Much later, the autistic child has a spontaneous tantrum over what appears to be nothing at all, or simply runs away to avoid being drawn into a social encounter. But, Kanner stressed, autistic aloneness is not the same as extreme shyness, nor does it refer to physical aloneness; rather it describes a pronounced emotional separation from what others are doing and saying and feeling.

Only about 50 percent of autistic children master ordinary speech, usually with significant delay. Some, like Jasmine, choose to communicate solely by the written word because they find that conversation draws them into exchanges that are too confusing for their fragile selves to bear. If they do speak, they may not use pronouns like *I* and *me* but rather they describe their own actions and feelings in the third person as though speaking of a stranger. Further contributing to the autistic child's aloneness is extreme sensitivity to sensations: some autistic children show signs of being physically pained by touch, noise, light, or smell. One mother has written, "Every time I give Nicky a kiss he wipes it away with his hand as if it were repulsive." Conversely, others seem to be strongly attracted to a limited range of sensations. Kanner also noted that these "alone" children often played happily with inanimate objects for hours. Presumably, objects are tolerated because they do not require emotional communication, do not demand socially correct behaviors, and can be played with on the child's terms.

The second characteristic, the *desire for sameness*, Dr. Kanner described as an anxious need to avoid outside change. He found that "the child's noises and motions and all his performances are . . . monotonously repetitious." Autistic children who do learn to speak tend to use very few words to express their thoughts. And they often speak in robotlike rhythms and tones, without emphasis and without distinguishing between the upward inflection of a question and the downward inflection of a declarative sentence. This is very different from the normal child who picks up rhythms and other vocal habits from his parents' speech even before his first birthday and begins babbling and forming human sounds, then words, then phrases, and finally whole sentences as his capacity grows.

Some autistic children will repeat the same phrases over and over, as though chanting. They may answer questions not with yes or no but by repeating the question. Similarly, they may express their desire for sameness by rocking back and forth, snapping their fingers, flapping their hands, or walking on their toes for days on end; or they may invent other seemingly meaningless motions that are uniquely their own. The need for sameness also extends to their physical environment. As the child with autism gets older, he or she makes it very clear that the placement of familiar furniture, the ordering of toys, the food he or she eats—almost anything that concerns personal space—must be "just so" to keep the peace. Small exceptions may trigger another tantrum or a siege of screaming over which the autistic child has no control. Closely related to this is a profound inability to switch attention from one activity to another.

Kanner's third marker—what he described as tiny *islands of ability* and what others call "splinter skills"—is demonstrated in one or more astonishing but narrowly focused splinter skills that the autistic child may possess. More than two centuries ago, Dr. Benjamin Rush, one of the very first Americans to investigate mental disorders, described the behavior of Thomas Fuller, an African slave. Rush, who knew nothing of autism, diagnosed the black man as mentally handicapped but noted that he possessed an uncanny skill at numerical calculation. When given a man's birth date, Fuller could instantly compute in his head the number of seconds the man had lived; he could even correct for leap years. In the late nineteenth century, Dr. J. Langdon Down, director of a London insane asylum, also studied a group of what modern scientists would describe as autistic people. In a lecture he delivered to the Medical Society of London, he described a group of "idiot savants," a French term meaning "possessed of unlearned skills," in his care. Each of the savants showed a singular ability in performing some feat of musical, artistic, mechanical, or mathematical memory without having received any formal training; a good many of these remarkable individuals appeared to be otherwise childlike, helpless, or even mentally deficient.

THE MANY FACES OF THE SAVANT

Today, we know that about one in ten people with autism has some savant skill. Those with musical ability most often reveal a gift for the piano, as is the case with Wisconsin's Leslie Lemke, born blind and otherwise mentally disabled, who can perform almost any music on the piano without ever having received training.[3] Savants with artistic ability can often draw or paint or sculpt to create near-perfect likenesses, though they may see their subject for the briefest moment. Alonzo Clemons, a sculptor who is otherwise severely disabled, has such a gift.[4] Savants with mechanical skills may be able to take apart and reassemble complex clockworks or other sorts of machinery without understanding how they operate. Others can memorize every detail of a map, discriminate smells of the most subtle differences, quote long strings of statistics, recall dates in history, or tell time to the minute without a watch, apparently by linking the passage of time to some internal body clock. Perhaps the best-known savant skill is the sort that Thomas Fuller displayed long ago: the ability to compute prime numbers or carry out some other kind of arithmetic exercise with lightening speed in the absence of any other math skill.

While no one can precisely explain the source of splinter skills, some theorists argue that the ability resides in the extraordinary focus that people with autism habitually bring to one sensation or object at a time by dint of their aloneness and their need for obsessive sameness. Others, noting that autistic people rarely engage in abstract thinking, believe that some of them develop a compensatory ability to harness "unconscious reckoning," a skill that these researchers suggest may exist at a more primitive level in all of us. (The ability of migratory animals to find their way over long distances may be a form of unconscious reckoning, too, as is the fairly widespread ability of seasoned travelers to know which way is north and so on.) The rest of us lose access to this primitive skill, they say, as our minds develop and we learn more subtle skills of sequential, logical, and symbolic thinking.

In 1988 actor Dustin Hoffman brought to the movie screen the fictional story of Raymond Babbitt, "The Rain Man." Babbitt was a young autistic man with a similar gift for numbers as well as spatial memorization. He had what we call a photographic memory, with which he was able to memorize phone books, maps, and other information and then scan them, "page by page" to find the particular data he needed at a later date. The Rain Man's story was closely modeled on the life of Joseph Sullivan, a high-functioning autistic savant of Huntington, West Virginia, whom Hoffman studied before making the film. Sullivan was born in 1960, the fifth of seven children of Drs. Ruth and William Sullivan. At age eighteen months, Joseph could put together a picture puzzle of the United States.[5] By age four he could draw maps of entire continents with all the countries and their capitals correctly located and spelled. Mixed in with these astonishing gifts, however, were the classic traits of autism—social withdrawal, a preoccupation with

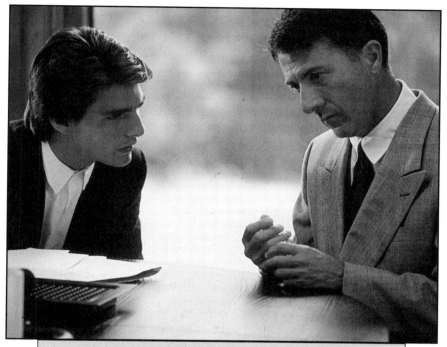

The 1988 film *Rain Man* explores the relationship between an ambitious young man (Tom Cruise, left) and his autistic older brother (Dustin Hoffman, right).

objects, compulsive ritual movements, extreme sensitivities to tactile and auditory stimulation, and inabilities to carry out many relatively simple activities. Joseph's speech was idiosyncratic in that he often spoke in a stream of recognizable words interspersed with favorite sounds, license plate numbers, and bits of memorization from the encyclopedia.

As Joseph grew older, he could multiply all sorts of large numbers in his head. Dr. Darrold Treffert, MD, who has written about Joseph, describes an exercise in which the young man was given the following thirty-six-number grid to study for two minutes:

$$
\begin{array}{cccccc}
6 & 2 & 4 & 8 & 4 & 9 \\
7 & 3 & 2 & 5 & 0 & 3 \\
4 & 8 & 9 & 3 & 4 & 3 \\
1 & 3 & 5 & 8 & 9 & 4 \\
5 & 7 & 2 & 8 & 4 & 2 \\
2 & 4 & 7 & 9 & 0 & 3
\end{array}
$$

Joseph was able to recall all thirty-six numbers correctly and in their original order; he did so in forty-three seconds.[6] To see just how amazing this is, try it yourself.

Unlike Raymond in the movie, who lives most of his life institutionalized, Joseph Sullivan has been able to live semi-independently in a group home and to hold a job. Through the efforts of activists like his mother, Ruth Sullivan, Joseph's community and many others have come to understand that despite their evident disabilities, many higher-functioning autistic people can make meaningful contributions to society if their limitations are understood and they are given suitable support. In Joseph's case, he shelves books in the public library, carrying out the kinds of highly repetitive and systematized tasks that particularly fit his capabilities.

THE MIND'S EYE

The majority of people with autism are unable to tell us much of their internal world or how they cope with being autistic. Fortunately, however, a few individuals have managed to pierce their aloneness to tell us quite a bit. One such exception is Temple Grandin. She has turned what most people perceive as autistic handicaps into skills that are valuable in her profession as a designer of livestock handling equipment for the cattle industry and as a teacher of Animal Science at Colorado State University. Dr. Grandin attributes her unique rapport with animals to her ability to focus all her concentration on their behaviors. She believes that she functions as well as she does because her parents recognized her disability early and were able to provide her with intense speech and behavioral training from the beginning.

Like Jasmine O'Neill and many other autistic people, Temple Grandin has always done most of her thinking in pictures. Grandin writes, "Words are like a second language to me. I translate both spoken and written words into full-color movies, complete with sound, which run like a VCR tape in my head. . . . The videos in my memory are always specific."[7] Thus, if someone tells her an anecdote about a cat, she can understand it only in terms of the particular cats she has known in her life; her mind must run through a sequence of those pictures beginning with the first cat she ever saw as a child to arrive at the notion of cats in general.

We know also that Grandin and autistic people like her tend to understand nouns more readily than other parts of speech, chiefly because nouns usually describe concrete things to which they can attach mental pictures. This is in contrast to prepositions like *of* and *to*; adjectives like *happy* and *sad*; verbs like *to do* or *to be*, all of which are abstract and elusive. This explains, too, why many colloquial phrases, slang words, and jokes are particularly baffling to the very literal mind of the person with autism.

Wendy Lawson, an Australian who has written extensively about the autistic experience, describes her difficulty understanding that a phrase like "hang around" translates as "wait" and not to being physically suspended; she cannot readily accept that "eat with your fork" has to do with which tool to use at the dining table rather than meaning "share your lunch with your fork." "I can remember my father telling me to 'make friends,'" says Lawson.[8] "I knew how to make a rice pudding, but I did not know how to 'make' friends." As an adult, Lawson still has difficulties going from specifics to generalized ideas and following conversations. But she knows herself well enough to realize that she cannot presume literal meanings in much of what she hears and reads. "Today I try to check out what is said. 'Is that something definite or just an idea?' I constantly ask questions, check out the rules and expectations. . . . Without formal outlines, boundaries and rules, I am flapping about like a fish out of water."

Grandin shares with many autistic people a wide range of "sensory dysfunctions," which simply means that she has a great deal of difficulty receiving, organizing, and interpreting information from her primary senses. Grandin's family initially thought that she was deaf, because she never seemed to respond to voices and was so late in learning speech. But Grandin explains that her state of inattentiveness then was really a matter of self-protection: She instinctively tuned out because the smallest sounds could sometimes cause her ears to "hurt like a dentist's drill hitting a nerve." She explains that noise was constantly assaulting her ears as though her "volume control [was] stuck on 'super loud' . . . [or] like an open microphone that picks up everything."[9] With so many confusing, conflicting signals coming at them, people with autism cannot process or "integrate" information meaningfully.

Errors in sensory integration can occur in many areas besides hearing, and they may cause unpredictable reactions ranging from revulsion to craving for more. Tactile hypersensitivity, for example, is almost certainly the explanation for why Grandin and the majority of autistic people cannot tolerate ordinary touch, as well as mild pain, pressure, and temperature variations. Grandin remembers that, as a child, she hungered to be touched but would nonetheless find herself pulling away. As she explains it, people either applied too much or too little pressure, never the "right" amount. To lessen her discomfort, she learned to crawl under the cushions of the family sofa or to wrap herself tightly in a blanket where she could control the pressure herself.

Then when she was about twelve and visiting her aunt's ranch, she chanced to attend a branding session down at the cattle pens. As the frightened animals were driven one by one into the narrow holding chute, she was amazed to see that once enclosed, they immediately calmed down. She reasoned that the side walls of the chute, by pressing on the cattle's bodies, somehow exerted a calming effect. She tried lying in the chute herself. When she, too, experienced relief, she built what she called her "Hug Box" or "Squeeze Machine." Made of two padded sideboards hinged near the bottom to form a V-shape, the holding box could be adjusted to create pressure. When she felt overwhelming anxiety, which was often the case in her teenage years, she could crawl into the space and press a simple lever that gradually brought the side boards together to create the deep pressure stimulation she needed.

Errors in tactile integration also explain why certain clothing, certain foods, having the face washed—all involving touch and texture—cause so much anxiety in many people with autism. Olfactory sensitivities may

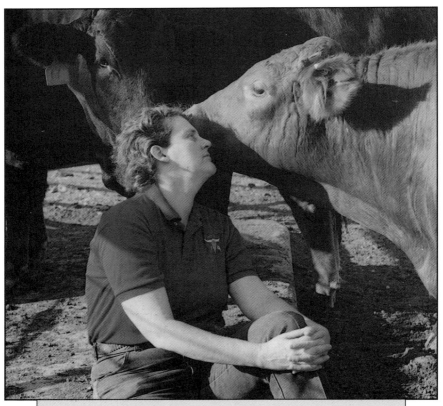

Dr. Temple Grandin has an affinity for animal behavior, a talent that is perhaps influenced by her own autistic experience.

excite tantrums or other reactions; many smells that the rest of us think of as "bad" because of their associations may conversely be "good" to the autistic person. Visual sensitivities can make flashing or bright lights intolerable. Vestibular reactivity—originating in the inner ear, or vestibule, and affecting movement, balance, and positioning of the head—can make some autistic children unusually fearful of swings, elevators, slides, stairs, and ramps. Other children with autism exhibit a seemingly inexhaustible need to overstimulate this sensory center, whirling and twirling, jumping and spinning, to the total exhaustion of those around them.

Proprioceptive or kinesthetic hypersensations—initiated in muscles, joints, and tendons and essential to coordinating posture and movement—are still another category of sensations that may trigger unusual reactions. They are probably the root cause of the autistic child's slowness in crawling and walking, their general clumsiness in using their hands and feet, their difficulty in feeding and in dressing themselves, their odd body posturing, and their tendency to fall down often.

Not surprisingly, autistic children may demonstrate different needs from hour to hour and from week to week, being constantly in motion and impulsive at one moment and exhausted and passive the next. Behavior problems often become worse in adolescence as children become more aware of their limitations and as their body chemistry is further complicated by the production of the many new hormones associated with the body's physical maturation.

CAUSES AND TREATMENTS

It is generally accepted now that autism, like many other behavioral and emotional disorders, has a biochemical basis. That leads researchers to believe that the production of certain neurotransmitters—chemical messengers that carry messages from one nerve cell in the brain to the next—was abnormal during fetal development. Whether the abnormality occurred as the result of environmental, infectious, metabolic, or genetic influences, or possibly some combination, is still unknown, but anything that caused too much or too little of certain proteins to be available at the time brain tissue was forming could be the explanation.

Indeed, in the years since it has been possible to look into living brains through positron emission technology (PET) scans and magnetic resonance imaging (MRI), researchers have observed subtle differences between the brain architecture of autistic children and that of children who function within normal ranges. Specifically, they find that the parts of the brain that control emotions and behavior—the limbic system—are either underdeveloped or overdeveloped. Tryptophan, an essential chemical involved in nerve cell communication, is one substance under investigation. Serotonin, which is synthesized from tryptophan, is another possible culprit. So far, the findings are intriguing but by no means conclusive. Genetic connections are also under the researchers' microscope. Though a role is definitely suspected, proving it is going to be extremely difficult, probably because multiple genes will turn out to be involved, and then only when some environmental factor is also present. Scientists estimate that in families with one autistic child, the risk of having a second child with the disorder is roughly 5 percent. That is higher than the general population, but certainly not on a par with disorders such as sickle cell anemia (Chapter 3) and Tay-Sachs (Chapter 5), which are clearly heritable.

There is currently no cure for autism. But appropriate medications and behavioral/educational therapies may moderate specific symptoms and promote relatively normal development and behavior; this is particularly so when the disorder is recognized early and treatments begun immediately. Unfortunately, autism has traditionally gone unrecognized for at least the first two to three years of a child's life, and even when parents and doctors begin to suspect that something is awry, misdiagnosis often leads them to apply the wrong treatments for some time. In this way precious time is lost.

Recent findings by Dr. Philip Teitelbaum, a member of the National Academy of Sciences and a psychologist at the University of Florida in Gainesville, give hope that in the near future it may be possible to recognize autism in infants as young as three months of age.[10] Dr. Teitelbaum approached parents whose children were later diagnosed as autistic and asked to see any videotapes they had of the children as infants. He noticed that he could pick out a subtle cluster of abnormalities in the way these babies rolled over, sat up, crawled, and walked, as compared with other babies who follow a rather consistent pattern of development. While he says that his discoveries are preliminary, if further study bears them out, it may be possible to intervene early enough in an autistic child's development to start intensive therapy when the brain is fairly elastic. As the brain of an infant is still constructing its basic network of nerves, physical therapy that corrects movement could actually stimulate new and corrective nerve growth to match.

Still other findings by researchers at the National Institute of Disorders and Stroke suggest another possible route to early diagnosis and treatment.[11] It involves the presence of four biochemical markers in blood that may be predictors of autism. One is a protein known familiarly as VIP, a kind of master molecule involved in the formation of brain tissue, which was found at abnormally high levels in blood samples of children who later developed autism. (For the past twenty years, California has banked blood samples of one in seven randomly selected newborns each year as part of ongoing epidemiological studies. Going back to these stored samples, it has been possible to compare the newborn blood of normal children with those of children who were later diagnosed as autistic.)

Meanwhile, educational/behavioral therapies are used to train today's generation of autistic children in the kinds of skills that will make them able to fit into their community more readily. Temple Grandin, for example, is able to interpret others' body language and tone of voice, not subconsciously, as most of us do, but by having diligently memorized what the cues mean. (She has thus committed to memory that a certain set of facial expressions that we call a smile means one thing and that other expressions—a frown, grimace, smirk, etc.—are fairly reliable cues to other feelings among people she deals with.) These days, high-functioning children with autism may also be exposed to training videos and interactive "social stories" by which they are read simple short stories and made to practice appropriate behaviors. Music therapy is also used in their speech training. Music is nonverbal; as autistic children often show considerable sensitivity to music even in the absence of speech, it can be an effective way to draw them into singing words first and then building speech upon the same patterns.

Drug interventions range from medications that reduce anxiety and hyperactivity to drugs that prevent epileptic seizures—roughly one third of autistic people experience occasional seizures, especially during adolescence. Secretin, a gastric hormone that has been used to treat the gastrointestinal problems that often accompany autism, was briefly hailed as reducing other autistic symptoms as well. It now seems less effective than originally hoped, though further studies continue.

The indications that autism may be on the increase in the United States and elsewhere has led some people to believe that environmental factors, including toxic substances in the air and water, as well as childhood vaccines may be a trigger for autism. In one highly publicized investigation, the CDC examined the public water supply and various other environmental chemicals found in Brick Township, New Jersey, after receiving reports of a startling cluster of autism cases—36 children born in 1998 alone in a population of 72,000. The CDC was able to verify that all the children were autistic according to the classic diagnostic criteria, but investigators were not able to pinpoint any environmental causes. The study has, however, drawn attention to the fact that scientific comparisons with national norms are not really possible as so little epidemiological data has been collected elsewhere to date. To rectify this situation and to pursue other discoveries into the causes and treatment of the entire spectrum of autistic disorders, the NIH is lately committing nearly $50 million annually to research in this area.[12]

ASPERGER SYNDROME

Asperger syndrome (AS) is part of the autism spectrum. AS children are often very bright and function at a higher level than other autistic children. Notably they usually develop language skills approaching that of normal youngsters, and they can often be mainstreamed in school. But owing to their focus on one piece of information at a time, they are sometimes misdiagnosed as having attention deficit disorder (ADD).

Not until 1994 did they enter medical diagnostic manuals as a group all their own.

Despite their ability to talk and use language, youngsters with AS lack the critical ability to read social cues and gestures, so they have great difficulty participating in conversations. When they do join in, their talk is usually very stilted and formal and focused on some set of facts with which they tend to be obsessed. For this reason Asperger syndrome is sometimes called "the little professor's disease." But youngsters with AS, according to Tony Attwood, a clinical psychologist who has studied them, can also take genuine pleasure in what they are doing and their excitement can "override all conventional codes of conduct. . . . [producing] a delirious state of euphoria that nothing else can compare with."[13]

Young Derek Preuss, for example, talks obsessively about game shows to the exclusion of all else; given the opportunity he will watch them constantly on TV, and when he talks about them it is as "game show host" to the "contestants" around him.[14] Similarly, Mikki Herbert has a passion for washing machines and dryers. Chad Mearhoff is single-minded in his interest in trains. And Darius McCollum, now thirty-five, has been incapacitated by his fixation on subways for decades, though only recently has anyone considered the possibility that his behavior has some explanation other than willful mischief. McCollum, who comes from a poor family and was not diagnosed as having AS until very recently, has been arrested and jailed nineteen times since 1981 for impersonating New York City transit employees and commandeering trains. His mother recalls that Darius was a very bright but unusual child from an early age. By five he had memorized the city's vast subway system and could provide directions to any point in the city. He also knew the specifications of particular trains and their schedules. She also remembers sadly that he was constantly picked on in school, had little success in making friends, and that the school psychologist found him "neurotic . . . insecure . . . with low self-esteem and grandiose ideas." As for Darius, he just wishes the transit authority would hire him. "To tell the truth, it would be a lot easier."[15]

Chapter Three

BAD BLOOD

SICKLE CELL ANEMIA AND OTHER BLOOD DISORDERS

Sickle cell anemia is a rare inherited blood disorder. It takes its name from the abnormally shaped red blood cells found in the bloodstream. The usually round, squishy, and smooth-flowing cells that transport hemoglobin molecules to every part of the body are altered to become long, pointed, and somewhat rigid sickle or crescent shaped. The malformed cells, instead of sliding through the vessels uneventfully, tend to snag on each other. They clump together, particularly in the capillaries, which are so small in diameter that cells can pass through them only in single file. Such blockages prevent the oxygen from being delivered and the adjacent tissue cannot function. This leads to intermittent and excruciatingly painful "crises" that require immediate treatment, usually including hospitalization. But there is a still larger price to be paid. Over the long term, the sickle cells perish faster than the body can replace them,

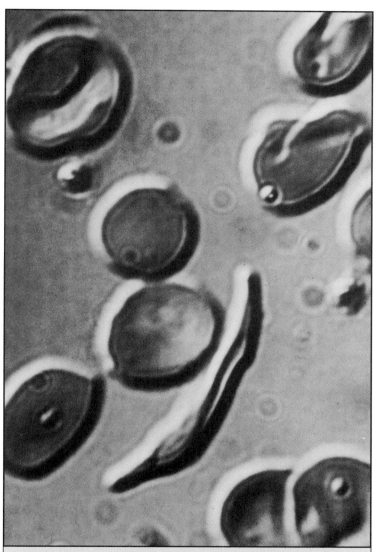

A sickle blood cell surrounded by normal blood cells. Its elongated shape prevents the sickle cell from moving smoothly through the bloodstream.

and this leads to systemwide oxygen starvation. Symptoms include headaches, dizziness, fatigue, muscle cramps, joint pain, shortness of breath, chest pain, pale tongue and lips, delayed puberty, nosebleeds, and jaundice. The disease is generally progressive as damage to the body's many organs—especially the spleen and liver—becomes cumulative. Until recent times, sickle cell disorder was almost always fatal in childhood. Improving methods of diagnosis and treatment have made it possible for more individuals with the disorder to live well into adulthood.

Sickle cell is primarily a genetic disease of blacks today, though it also appears in a tiny percentage of people from the Mediterranean basin—Italy, Sardinia, and Greece, as well as in people of Indian and Middle Eastern heritage. It is a *congenital* disorder in that it is present at birth and can be detected immediately through blood tests. It is also *unifactorial* in that it is a result of a defect in one gene controlling the production of a particular essential protein. And it is *autosomal recessive* in that it becomes an active disorder only when both parents are *carriers* of the defective gene. Individuals who carry a single copy of the recessive gene do not develop full-blown sickle cell disease, though they may be mildly anemic; they are sometimes referred to as being *heterozygous* for sickle cell. However, should they join with a parenting partner who is also an asymptomatic carrier, they have a one-in-four chance of producing a child with full-blown sickle cell; the child is referred to as being *homozygous* for the trait. By the same classic laws of Mendelian inheritance, that offspring also has a two-in-four chance of becoming a carrier and a one-in-four chance of inheriting neither the trait nor the disease. The risk is the same for each child of the same parents, so it is theoretically possible that several siblings might have active sickle cell anemia, but it is also possible that none will.

In some parts of Africa, the sickle cell trait is present in 40 percent of the general population, with the frequency varying somewhat according to geography. This almost certainly reflects the historic isolation of some tribal groups who have tended to marry largely within their own groups for hundreds if not thousands of years. In the United States, the incidence of the sickle cell trait is considerably lower—about 9 percent—but that still works out to be about 1 in 350 African-American newborns for a total number of cases running around 90,000. Sickle cell is also found widely in the Caribbean and in parts of Central and South America where African blacks were transported during the era of the slave trade.

GENETIC ORIGINS

Geneticists believe that sickle cell originated, perhaps as a single gene mutation, in Neolithic times, roughly 12,000 years ago. They further postulate that it began in the Arabian peninsula, but that as climatic changes caused the original "cradle" of sickle cell to turn increasingly dry and desertlike, sickle cell carriers migrated east, west, north, and south to more habitable areas. In the process, they carried the mutant gene to India, the eastern Mediterranean, and Africa, and most particularly to equatorial West Africa. The peoples there have many names for the disorder, most of them thought to be onomatopoeic imitations of the sounds made by children in pain. The Ga people of modern day Ghana, for example, call sickle cell anemia *Chwecheechwe*, while their countrymen the Fante call it *Nwiiwii*. The Ewe speak of it as *Nuidudui*; the Twi know it as *Ahututo*.

Not until the twentieth century was any scientific attention given to the causes and character of sickle cell anemia. The first to begin asking questions was Dr. James B. Herrick (1861–1954), a Chicago heart specialist. In 1910, Herrick chanced to examine an anemic twenty-year-old student from the West Indies. Herrick reported "peculiar elongated and sickle-shaped" red cells in the young man's blood and tentatively associated what he saw with the anemia. "Sickling" was described in great detail seven years later by another American, V. E. Emmel (1878–1928), who treated a black woman with severe anemia and leg ulcers. Emmel went on to examine the woman's father's blood and was puzzled to find that a small proportion of his red cells also sickled but only under laboratory conditions and without causing anemia in the individual. The father was almost certainly a carrier. Five years later, Emmel's colleague J. G. Huck explored the incidence of sickle cell within families and began to sketch the evidence of a hereditary link. By this time it was also recognized that the sickling of red cells occurred when the oxygen concentration in the blood was lower than normal.

The next big breakthroughs came after World War II. In 1949 the American chemist Linus Pauling and his coworkers traced the sickling specifically to abnormal hemoglobin, which they called hemoglobin S, for "sickle." Further study of hemoglobin S revealed that it was far less soluble than normal hemoglobins A and F. In fact when hemoglobin S is packed tightly inside the red cells, it forms tiny crystals that bulge through the membranes to distort cells into their characteristic sickle shapes. In 1956, Dr. Vernon Ingram, working at

Britain's famed Cavendish Laboratory, isolated the specific abnormality—a mutation in a single gene that produces the abnormal protein underlying the blood disorder. This, in turn, has led to our current knowledge of sickle cell anemia.

Epidemiologists, the scientists who study the geographic distributions of diseases, noticed that the most pronounced pockets of sickle cell disease were virtually identical with those areas in which two other factors were present: the incidence of yam cultivation and the scourge of malarial infection. For a time, epidemiologists pursued both leads as possible causative factors, but yams as a dietary staple were eventually exonerated as mere coincidence. But the connection between sickle cell and malaria did turn out to play a surprising role.

British investigators knew that, at the time, at least 90 percent of individuals who had active sickle cell anemia died at a relatively young age. This would ordinarily lead over time to the dying out of the lethal gene if it had no redeeming qualities. Yet in treating African children in jungle hospitals, they began to notice that, unlike the other children who came in for various medical treatments, virtually all the youngsters brought in with severe infantile malaria lacked the sickling trait. Malaria, which is a parasitic disease transmitted by the anopheles mosquito and a predominant cause of chronic sickness and death in Central Africa, also happens to live in the bloodstream. From this they deduced that sickle cell conferred some survival advantage over malaria that counterbalanced its obvious disadvantage.

Further study has shown that when malarial parasites invade the bloodstream, they tend to be swallowed up in the sickling cells where, because sickle cells have a shorter life span than normal red blood cells, they die before they can reproduce and multiply. For that reason, those who are sickle cell carriers but do not themselves have the disorder are protected from contracting full-blown malaria; they consequently tend to live longer, to be healthier generally, and to have the opportunity to produce more children than those who do not have the sickling trait. (They also risk having sickle cell offspring if they mate with a second carrier, of course.) Having this compensatory characteristic is, however, of no positive value in the United States or anywhere else that antimalarial medicines and programs are in place. So it's safe to say that sickle cell anemia has only a very clear downside in the modern western world.

DETECTION

Routine blood counts commonly performed in doctors' offices do not disclose the presence or absence of the sickle cell trait. It takes a special test, called "hemoglobin electrophoresis," to make a determination. Electrophoresis is based on the fact that the differing proteins that make up hemoglobin carry different-strength electrical charges; consequently, they travel at different rates through an electric field, their particles forming "bands" that separate toward one end or the other in the field. The bands appear as slight variations in the refraction, or bending, of a light ray as it passes through them. In 1987 the NIH recommended that all newborns, regardless of ethnic or racial background or country of origin, be tested for sickle cell disease at birth. Most states, though not all, have followed those recommendations, for it is widely recognized that the earlier a child is diagnosed with the disorder, the higher the survival rate. The test is performed by taking a tiny blood sample from the baby's heel using a simple needle prick. Parents whose infant is diagnosed with sickle-cell disease can then be offered information on follow-up care and treatment, advice that is particularly important during the first seven years of life when symptoms may not routinely reveal themselves but when overwhelming and potentially fatal bacterial infections are possible.

Genetic testing is another means of detection. Genetic testing involves the analysis of genes and related products to determine if some alteration from the normal genetic code is causing, or is likely to cause, a specific disease or condition. The tests are carried out by a skilled geneticist who begins by examining the family history of both parents for evidence of diseases in past and present generations; further examination often follows using the appropriate chemical or DNA analysis. There are several circumstances in which genetic testing may be justifiably used, but it is almost always done under careful scrutiny and with great regard for the privacy of the individuals involved. Quite apart from what aid it may give individuals in making certain life decisions, the information gained can reach potential employers or health insurers and cause the individual with a positive finding of one disorder or another to be rejected. While there are laws against discrimination in employment and health insurance, such laws are difficult to enforce.

Because sickle cell anemia involves a single mutant gene in a well-defined minority population, it was one of the first disorders to be identified through genetic testing and forecasting. An at-risk couple wanting to know in advance their probability of producing a child with full-blown sickle cell disorder has the option to seek genetic counseling for the answer. And if they find that they are both carriers, they may decide that they do not wish to risk producing children who might have the disorder or the trait. Alternatively, genetic testing also makes it possible during the first four months after conception for a carrier couple to discover whether they have passed on the one-in-four disorder to their unborn child. The evidence can be picked up in amniocentesis, a diagnostic procedure in which a small amount of amniotic fluid is withdrawn from the sac surrounding the fetus in utero (in the womb) and examined to detect fetal abnormalities. Testing for birth defects in utero is seen by some ethicists as raising the sensitive issue of eugenics and is consequently a hotly debated topic within and without the medical community.

The term *eugenics* was coined in the late nineteenth century from a Greek word meaning "well born." It was proposed at a time when the nature of genes and what they did was still unknown. Eugenicists thought of "well-born qualities" or traits as describing characteristics such as physical beauty, intelligence, honesty, and artistic ability, and they set out to encourage those with qualities that they deemed desirable to reproduce more prolifically. At the same time, the eugenicists also sought to discourage people with qualities they deemed "undesirable" to produce fewer or no children. The seeds of eugenics took hold, spreading rapidly wherever economic and racial intolerance also existed. By the end of the first decade of the twentieth century, it was used as an argument for restricting immigration in some places and even for legalized involuntary sterilization of people thought to be socially undesirable. The Nazi death camps of World War II were the ultimate expression of this kind of human engineering gone mad, and certainly no civilized society today would condone such practices for the purposes of "improving" the human race.

Since no medical intervention is as yet available to correct sickle cell disorder in the fetus, the only presumed value in testing for the disorder before birth is to be able to abort if an abnormality is found. And it is that ability to pick and choose among fetuses on the basis of a detectable genetic defect that makes some people fear a "new eugenics" in the making.

TREATMENT

Treating a child for sickle cell disorder is largely a matter of keeping the child as healthy as possible and treating symptoms early. Because of the high risk of infections, children with sickle cell disorder should be examined frequently and, in addition to all the usual childhood immunizations, they should receive annual flu shots and be vaccinated against pneumonia, to which they are unusually prone. Because dehydration is an ongoing concern, they must also drink quantities of fluids each day, and they should be extra careful to avoid emotional or physical stress, including traveling at high altitudes, particularly when they are experiencing breathing problems due to oxygen deprivation. Good nutrition, including folic acid, a vitamin essential to producing red blood cells, is also urgently recommended. Mild pain can be treated with over-the-counter painkillers (analgesics) such as nonsteroidal anti-inflammatory drugs (NSAIDs), excepting aspirin, which children's stomachs do not tolerate well.

Sickle cell crises, which are acute (short term), extremely painful, and serious events, require rapid response, because the pain is an indication of cell death that must be halted to avoid permanent damage. Oxygen therapy, blood transfusions, and powerful narcotic drugs, often administered in the hospital, are the usual first line of defense. Adding to the pain of such crises, many adult sickle cell patients find that it is often difficult to get the help they need for their pain because of the medical community's reluctance to prescribe narcotics medicinally. Adults who rush to a hospital emergency room seeking relief from agonizing chest and joint pain frequently report that they meet only hostility. Medical personnel who do not know these patients and have little experience in treating acute sickle cell cases, regard them as drug addicts who are faking pain symptoms just to "get a fix." Complications of sickle cell disorder, including leg sores, opportunistic infections, organ failure, and stroke, are some of the other associated risks that the individual with sickle cell and his or her caregivers must be ready to recognize and treat. Lastly, emotional support from friends and family is essential to anyone bearing the brunt of this difficult and sometimes discouraging disorder.

Until recently, there were few targeted drugs available to ease particular symptoms, but in 1998 the FDA approved the drug hydroxyurea (Droxia) for reducing the frequency of painful episodes in adults. (Hydroxyurea was already approved for treating certain cancers, but it had to be clinically tested and approved all over again to be prescribed for this second use.) Other orphan drug applications are now in progress and may be approved in the very near future. At the same time, research into finding more fundamental ways to protect against the ravages of sickle cell continue.

Experimental treatments currently focus on the events that cause the red cells to sickle in the first place. The most promising to date is bone-marrow transplantation. Marrow, the soft material found at the center of bones, produces stem cells; these are the precursor cells from which all other cells of more specialized nature grow, including red blood cells. The intent of this high-tech therapy is to destroy the sickle cell patient's diseased bone marrow and stem cells and replace them with the marrow and stem cells of a healthy donor, thereby wiping out the sickle cell disorder altogether. But, like any form of transplantation, the risks are very high and the success rate still far less than medical science finds acceptable. Only about 1 percent to 2 percent of children with sickle cell are even considered viable candidates.

Still another avenue of treatment lies in gene therapy, or gene transfer therapy as it is now more properly known. The idea behind gene transfer therapy is that desirable genetic material can be delivered into living cells where it will recombine at the right place on the right chromosome to produce normal cells that will then begin to reproduce and provide a permanent change in the individual's genetic makeup. The first human experiment of this kind was launched in 1990 under NIH supervision, and for a time scientists hailed recombinant gene therapy as the bold new answer to hundreds if not all genetic disorders. Time has shown, however, that this is far more difficult and dangerous to achieve than was originally imagined; effective and consistently reliable treatment by this method is now considered to be several years away.

HEMOPHILIA AND OTHER BLOOD DISORDERS

Another devastating category of hereditary blood diseases is hemophilia. A very ancient disease, historians can trace the recognition of hemophilia in Old Testament law: Any family that had two sons die during circumcision was formally exempted from having any more sons circumcised on account of their

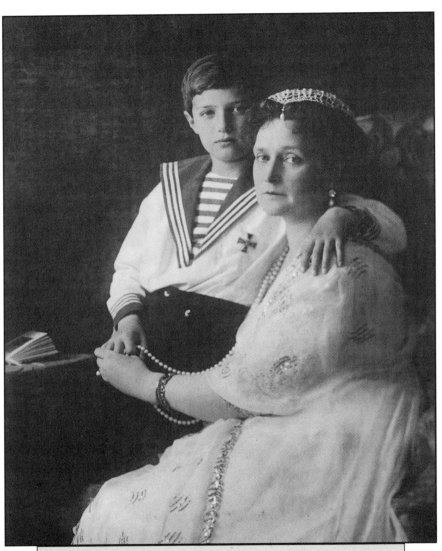

Alexandra, the empress of Russia, with her son, the young czarevitch, Alexei. The boy suffered from hemophilia, a condition he inherited from his mother.

belonging to a family of "bleeders." Hemophilia was mentioned again in medical texts dating from the second century A.D. And it has figured in the royal succession of several European monarchies, for which reason it is sometimes popularly known as "the disease of kings." It is now thought that hemophilia was carried by no less a figure than Queen Victoria of England, and that through two of her granddaughters it passed to the monarchies of Spain and Russia.

All forms of hemophilia, though they vary widely in severity, have the same basic symptom, which is the blood's inability to clot properly. This leaves individuals at high risk of bleeding, internally and externally, after even a minor cut or bruise. The fault lies in the interaction of two blood factors—the platelets and a fibrous protein—that normally work together to seal wounds within seconds of injury but that are lacking or deficient here. Hemophilia A and hemophilia B are both X-linked forms of the disorder, affecting boys only but passed on by unaffected carrier mothers; A occurs in about 1 in 5,000 and B in about 1 in 40,000 male births. Von Willebrand's disease, yet another form of hemophilia, occurs in 1 in 20,000 to 30,000 births and is divided indiscriminately between boys and girls.

Severe forms of hemophilia are treated with replacement clotting factor, which is injected periodically in concentrated form. For many years, the clotting factor could be distilled only from human blood, making it a difficult and unreliable source. (Contaminated blood was responsible for the widespread transmission of AIDS to many hemophiliacs back in the 1970s and 1980s, before careful screening for the HIV virus was instituted.) Today several pharmaceutical companies produce recombinant and/or wholly artificial forms of clotting factor as a viable substitute.

The term *anemia*, used in the context of sickle cell disorder, turns up in several other rare and not-so-rare blood disorders. The rare *heritable anemias* include thalassemia and Fanconi's anemia. Thalassemia is largely confined to people of Mediterranean descent and is characterized by red blood cells that are uncommonly fragile and thin and consequently short-lived. Fanconi's anemia, named for the Swiss physician who first described it in 1927, causes bone marrow failure, eventually resulting in leukemia, other cancers, and death by the fifth year if a bone-marrow transplant from a perfectly matched sibling cannot be made. From birth, children with Fanconi's anemia have a pronounced reduction not only in blood platelets but in all kinds of white blood cells as well, together with extensive other congenital abnormalities. Though rare in the general population, it appears in notable concentrations in people of eastern Jewish heritage (see Chapter 5 for more).

The more common *deficiency anemias* are due to insufficiencies of a certain vitamin or mineral in the body and are often reversible these days with dietary changes or supplements. Iron-deficiency anemia, for example, often happens in children, pregnant and menstruating women, people with chronic bleeding ulcers, or in individuals on weight reduction diets, when their ordinary nutritional intake is not enough to keep up with normal iron loss. Pernicious anemia is a blood disease in which the red blood cells are normal in composition and architecture but few in number. It is caused by a lack of vitamin B12 in the diet or by the inability of the intestine to absorb the vitamin because of the lack of a certain protein that aids normal absorption; it, too, can usually be treated by diet or periodic injections of the missing vitamin. Folic acid anemia occurs occasionally in pregnant women, alcoholics, and the elderly due to dietary deficiencies and can be treated with folic acid supplements.

Hemolytic anemias occur when the rate at which red blood cells are destroyed increases beyond the body's ability to replace them. An allergic reaction to some drugs and malarial infection are two possible causes. Hemolytic anemia of the newborn can occur as a result of Rh incompatibility between mother and child and the resulting destruction of red blood cells by hostile antibodies. A vaccine administered as part of prenatal care is the standard preventive. *Aplastic anemias* are traceable to a decrease in the production of all types of blood cells by the bone marrow. The cause is sometimes unknown, but usually exposure to radiation, chemotherapy, or toxic chemicals such as benzene or arsenic is found to be the triggering event. Regular blood transfusions are usually the only effective treatment to maintain strength and to fight infection.

Chapter Four

OF LITTLE PEOPLE AND BRITTLE BONES

RARE BONE AND CONNECTIVE TISSUE DISORDERS

There are roughly three hundred rare bone and connective tissue disorders that can cause youngsters to grow to greater or lesser than normal stature. In this chapter, we will look more closely at two of them: achondroplasia, or dwarfism, and osteogenesis imperfecta, or break bone disorder.

Achondroplasia (*chondro* refers to cartilage, *plasia* to formation, and the prefix *a* indicates "a lack") occurs in all races and with equal frequency in males and females. Like so many rare diseases, this condition is traceable to a single chemical change or genetic mutation that occurs at conception. Normally, the fetus goes through a series of transformations in which soft cartilage develops and is gradually replaced by bone. But in achondroplasia the foundation cartilage is defective, giving rise to stunted bone development. Consequently, the individual grows to less than fifty-five inches in height at maturity; indeed, some affected persons may not exceed twenty-four inches. Currently in the United States alone there are some 10,000 individuals living with achondroplasia; estimates of the numbers of babies born each year with this condition vary, but according to the Greenburg Center, a research facility that is devoted to studying and treating skeletal dysplasias, at Johns Hopkins Medical Center, the frequency range is between 1 in 26,000 and 1 in 40,000.[1] In nine out of ten instances, the underlying mutation is spontaneous, with the parents being of normal stature. However, as the mutation is dominant, a person with achondroplasia has a 50 percent chance of producing offspring with the same condition. When both parents are short-statured, they have a one in four likelihood of having a child with "double dominant" achondroplasia, a genetic inheritance that is almost always fatal shortly after birth.

THE SHORT STORY

Achondroplasia often manifests itself visibly, even in the newborn. The head and trunk may be close to normal size, but the extremities will be subtly shorter in proportion. (Proportionate dwarfism—where the individual's anatomical parts are in the same size relation to each other found in a normal individual—is often the result of a hormonal deficiency and may be treated medically.) Facial abnormalities may also be apparent in achondroplasia, with the forehead prominent, the jaw protruding, and the central portion of the face receding more than normal. As the infant grows, these characteristics tend to become exaggerated. The teeth come in misaligned because of crowding. The long bones of the legs become bowed rather than straight. The arms cannot be extended fully because elbows are twisted slightly and hands and feet are short and broad. The spine and pelvis may also have an exaggerated tilt and the buttocks are extended. The ligaments that hold the skeletal bones together are looser than normal, giving the impression of double-jointedness.

Children with achondroplasia typically reach motor development milestones such as good head control, crawling, and walking later than otherwise normal children simply because their musculature takes additional time to grow strong enough to compensate for their disproportionate parts. Eventually, however, these youngsters usually catch up, developing agility and considerable strength, as well as maturing sexually and having an otherwise normal life span. "Little People," as they generally prefer to be known, have the same distribution of clever, bright, and ambitious people as the rest of the population. Indeed, it is a matter of historical record that in the prescientfic era, dwarfs were more often than not thought of as specially prized individuals. Their childlike size coupled with their adult intelligence conferred upon them the appearance of almost divine wisdom in some cultures, and they were often retained as advisors and entertainers in the entourages of Egyptian and Roman dignitaries. In medieval and Renaissance Europe, Little People were especially favored at the courts of Spain, Germany, and the Italian city states, and in eighteenth- and nineteenth-century Russia, their presence in the households of tsarist noblemen was considered to bring good fortune.

In more recent times, P. T. Barnum hired several dwarfs to perform in his American Museum. Forty-inch, seventy-pound Charles Stratton of Bridgeport,

Connecticut, became far and away the most famous. Later known as "General Tom Thumb," he went on tour at the age of five. He eventually married another Barnum performer, the thirty-two-inch Lavinia Warren. Their elaborately staged wedding held in New York City in 1863 was reported in detail around the world. (Both Stratton and Warren appear to have had hypochondroplasia, a variant on achondroplasia in which the body is somewhat closer to normal proportions despite short stature.) Acting roles continue to offer occasional opportunities to Little People, among them the 124 dwarfs who were cast to play the roles of Munchkin villagers in the 1939 film classic, *The Wizard of Oz*. In 1999, Little Person Verne Troyer costarred with Mike Meyers in the film *Austin Powers: The Spy Who Shagged Me*.

LIVING WITH ACHONDROPLASIA

The gene for achondroplasia was discovered in 1994 by a team of researchers at the University of California at Irvine. In succeeding years, the sites for many other even rarer forms of dwarfism were also isolated. The discoveries came more rapidly than anyone had anticipated, creating a sudden and unexpected set of medical, social, and ethical dilemmas that demanded serious consideration. Particularly unsettled were members of the Little People of America (LPA), an organization set up in 1957 to provide peer support, as well as to educate the public and dispel myths on behalf of LPs. On the one hand, they could see a real advantage in couples with achondroplasia being able to identify a fetus with double dominant syndrome. Individuals with achondroplasia are, for obvious reasons, often drawn to each other during their dating years and when they marry

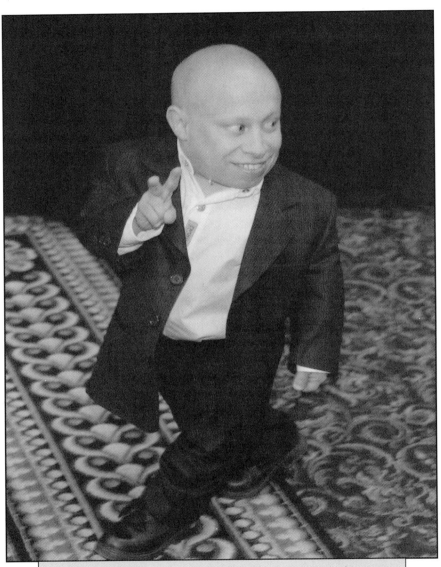

Actor Verne Troyer, the celebrated "Mini-Me" character of the popular Austin Powers movie sequel they have a heightened likelihood of choosing a partner of similar stature. But as prospective parents, they run a 25 percent risk of losing their offspring at or shortly after birth, a heartache that very few couples would readily endure if they had the means to choose early termination and to begin again. (By the classic Mendelian equation, the same couple has a 75 percent chance of producing a healthy child, either an LP child like themselves or a full-sized child.)

Many members of the LPA worry that the same screening techniques may, however, become part of a routine package of genetic screening tests that all expectant mothers will seek soon after conception. If so, they fear that it will become too easy to abort any fetus showing evidence of any anomaly at all. Further, they anticipate that at some point in medical progress, it may also become possible to snip out and replace any mutant gene with a normal gene in utero. As the leadership of the LPA has written on this matter, they feel they have come too far in achieving self-acceptance, pride, community, and culture to see others take away the opportunity for life of many like themselves without due consideration. "We as short statured individuals are productive members of society," they declare. "We value the opportunity to contribute a unique perspective to the diversity of our society."[2] They do not favor eradicating future generations of people like themselves just because it becomes medically possible.

What are the health challenges LPs live with? LPs may have secondary medical issues arising out of their skeletal dysplasia. In childhood, the most frequent difficulty is with ear infections (otitis media) and sleep apnea (interrupted breathing during sleep), owing to the peculiar shape, size, and tilt of certain internal bony structures involved in hearing and breathing. Many LPs need orthopedic bracing, particularly of their legs, during the growing years, when knock-knees, bowing, or a configuration termed "windswept," in which both legs bend in the same way as if some great force were pushing sideways against them, can develop. Complex dental work may be necessary to improve the alignment of teeth and jaws. Extremely delicate surgery may be required to enlarge the rigid passage (foramen magnum) between the base of the brain stem and the top of the spinal column, where a pinched spinal cord can cause excruciating pain and numbness. Even when an LP escapes most of these consequences, it's not unusual as an adult to develop chronic back pain stemming from the curvature of the spine and resulting compression of the spinal cord or nerve roots. Advanced orthopedic surgery may be necessary to alleviate discomfort.

Even when achondroplasia does not cause major medical problems, LPs face many obstacles to living comfortable, independent lives. Though opinions vary within the LP community as to whether theirs is a disability or not, even otherwise healthy short-statured persons qualify for special considerations under the Americans for Disabilities Act. Many of the obstacles are external, or "environmental" as they term them. Short-statured people must learn to navigate in a world that is not set up physically for people whose bodies are significantly different. Everything from clothing to furniture to phone booths to automobiles and household appliances are oversized for them, necessitating adaptive equipment to make them workable. Theirs is a life of step stools and extension pedals and make-do. Such simple things as door knobs and wall light switches, public toilets and ATM machines, musical instruments

Looking at Labels

The modern terminology used in describing persons of short stature is somewhat complex, in large part because so many of the old labels were used indiscriminately as words of insult or ridicule. Today, a person with achondroplasia generally prefers to be described as a "dwarf," "Little Person," or LP. Most LPs consider the term *midget* offensive, though it has as well a secondary use as a descriptor of small-statured people of normal proportions. The term *pygmy* applies to members of any human group whose males grow on average to fifty-nine inches or less as a normal characteristic of their racial group; the best-known pygmies are nomadic hunter-gatherers who live in scattered parts of the Central African rain forest. *Cretin* is an obsolete and offensive term for persons who have congenital hypothyroidism, resulting in insufficient thyroid secretion, diminished growth, and mental retardation.

Having said all this, it is also important to remember that most people, whatever their circumstance, would rather not be labeled at all but be thought of as individuals with their own unique personalities, abilities, needs, and desires.

and computer keyboards are hard to master; some devices specifically designed to promote safety—such as the air bags in cars—can be dangerous. Even keeping pace with others when walking can be exhausting due to the naturally shorter stride of the LP.

Short-statured people also have to live with the stereotypical attitudes toward shortness. People who would never be so cruel as to ridicule a person with physical scarring or a lost arm or leg can be very thoughtless when it comes to their treatment of short-statured individuals. This is particularly so during the school years when other children can taunt an LP mercilessly. Parents and others who are part of the LP's inner circle must be particularly sensitive to helping them develop a sense of self-worth in such a harsh environment. It was only a few years ago that the singer-composer Randy Newman performed what he thought was a very funny song called "Short People," but many people—most particularly LPs—were not amused.

CONTROVERSIAL TREATMENTS

Two treatments that have been developed to modify some of the symptoms of achondroplasia are not without controversy. The first is the use of growth hormones. While growth hormone supplements show some effect in increasing stature in the youngster under a year or so, it now appears that they simply speed up the growth process but make no change in the individual's mature stature.

The other intervention is limb lengthening surgery (LLS). First tried in Russia in the 1950s, it was introduced in the United States in the late 1980s and immediately divided the LP community into proponents, who see the functional advantages of being taller, and critics, who worry that it is being done for cosmetic purposes at the risk of long-term damage to nerves, muscle, and bone.

Gillian Mueller, who began the procedure in 1988 when she was thirteen, takes a distinctly different

74

view.[3] She underwent three years of treatment at the Maryland Center for Limb Lengthening and Reconstruction in Baltimore, under Dror Paley, MD, one of a handful of American experts in this technique. We will let Gillian describe what happened in her own words.

"That June, I had the first procedure on my tibias. Dr. Paley broke the bone just above my ankle and just below my knee and inserted several wires, which were attached to an external apparatus to hold the bone in place. A week later I began turning screws that would force the bone apart." Gradually, new bone tissue began to grow internally, filling the gap much as it does when a bone breaks in a natural fracture. But because the gap was continuously being enlarged by turning the external screws, the bone healed longer as it simultaneously filled the gap.

While Gillian's legs were being stretched, she kept busy with physical therapy routines by day. Nights were more difficult as she did not always sleep well. But the procedure was at no time particularly painful, nor was she troubled with any of the infections or other complications that sometimes occur. When both lower legs had been extended to near normal length, she underwent similar reconstruction on her upper legs and then on her arms. In all, she grew from roughly four feet tall to just over five feet.

Others of Dr. Paley's patients—and he and his codirector Dr. John Herzenberg have treated more than four thousand by now—have attained as much as fourteen additional inches. Given the relative newness of the procedure, it is still somewhat early to speak of life-long benefits and risks, but the majority of those who have undergone it speak enthusiastically of the results.

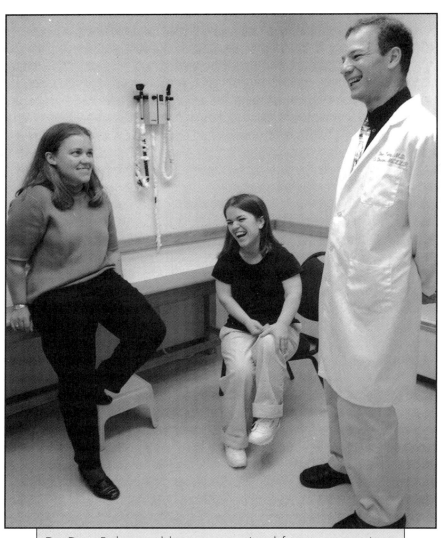

Dr. Dror Paley and his assistant (and former patient)
Gillian Mueller (left) chat with a teenage patient
during a follow-up exam. The youngster is undergoing
a limb lengthening procedure.

OSTEOGENESIS IMPERFECTA: HANDLE WITH CARE

It's Sunday evening at the emergency room (ER) of a community hospital in southern Illinois. Margaret and Evan O'Neil are talking excitedly to a policeman and a social worker in one of the examining cubicles. Nearby, two doctors finish setting and casting the arm of their four-year-old son, Peter. Neither the boy nor his parents can explain what caused the accident. They insist that he was simply playing with the family dog when he cried out in pain. The doctors, on the other hand, suspect physical abuse. Routine X rays have revealed not only a fresh fracture in Peter's lower arm but two earlier breaks in the wrist and upper arm in different stages of healing. They have consequently done what the law and their own ethical standards require, which is to alert the authorities to a possible problem. The social worker and the policeman, sharing their concern, tell the O'Neils that they may be charged with endangerment. Meanwhile, the authorities will take Peter, for his own safety, to stay with a foster family.

Sadly, scenes like this occur in ERs every day. And often the doctors and the others are justified in their actions. But as everyone involved will eventually learn, Peter is not the victim of child abuse. He is, rather, one of an estimated 20,000 to 50,000 people in the United States who have break bone disorder, or osteogenesis imperfecta (OI). OI is a genetic disorder involving the manufacture of collagen—the protein "scaffolding" that goes to construct bone and other connective tissues. The gene that instructs Peter's body to make collagen is sending faulty messages, with the result that the amount of collagen made is too little or is of poor quality. This causes Peter's bones to break rather easily, particularly in his young years when he is growing quickly.

Most people with osteogenesis imperfecta inherit it. Classed as an autosomal dominant disorder, it typically takes only a single copy of the disease gene received from either the mother or the father for OI to appear. The carrier parent has a fifty-fifty chance of passing the disorder to each of his or her children. Often the parent is not even aware of carrying the trait. But it is also possible for the condition to arise through a spontaneous genetic mutation; one in four individuals with OI is born into a family in which there is no history of brittle bones.

The condition varies widely in seriousness, with bones that bow and break being the common denominator in all types. But in Type I, the mildest and most common form, the vulnerabilities are greatest before puberty when physical growth is fastest, after which bones fracture with less frequency. Generally speaking, Type I children also grow to near normal height, though they may appear less tall than they are because of a tendency to have scoliosis, or curvature of the spine. (Two exceptionally short individuals with OI are Lin Yih-Chih of Taipei, Taiwan, who is twenty-seven inches tall, and Madge Bester of South Africa, who is twenty-six inches tall. They are currently listed in the *Guinness Book of World Records* as the shortest man and woman on earth.)

Other symptoms may include a bluish cast to the whites of the eyes, brittle teeth, loose joints, early hearing loss, a barrel-shaped chest, breathing problems, and frequent bruising from minor bumps. Ordinary activities like having a diaper changed or being burped can cause fracturing in an OI baby during his or her first months, particularly if the condition has not yet been recognized and the parents are not aware that they must handle their child with extraordinary delicacy.

Learning to crawl and then to walk are also dangerous times for the OI toddler, who may sustain multiple mild but fracturing bumps that may be the first telltale signs of the disease. By school age most children with OI have had more than enough opportunities to learn that they have to move through life with greater caution than their peers, though they can usually attend mainstream schools and look forward to a life of independence. Type II OI is the rarest form of all and it is frequently fatal at an early age because of the secondary problem of underdeveloped lungs and the child's vulnerability to respiratory distress.

MAKING IT BETTER

There is no cure for OI. Treatment these days focuses on repairing the fractures as often as they occur and keeping youngsters up and moving about as much as possible, rather than putting them in wheelchairs or slowing them down any more than is absolutely necessary. As orthopedic research makes quite clear, bones—even brittle bones—have a better chance at getting stronger, denser, more massive, through active use and weight bearing. Safe exercises and physical therapy are still the best medicine available. Especially helpful is therapeutic swimming; it exercises the whole body, but as the body is somewhat buoyant in water, stress on all parts of the skeletal system is lessened.

At one time, nutritional approaches were also widely followed. OI children were put on megadoses of calcium and magnesium, the basic building blocks of normal bone, together with growth hormones and calcitonin, a hormone that enhances the deposition of calcium and phosphate in bone. But though a generally nutritious diet continues to be recommended, as it is for all children, special diets are no longer considered particularly effective, and the hormones have been found to have detrimental side effects.

One class of drugs that has been found to show promising results is the bisphosphonates, currently approved for treating older women and men suffering from osteoporosis. These drugs—of which the best-known proprietary version is Fosamax—promote the absorption of available bone-building minerals. This makes bones denser and consequently stronger. To date, none of the drugs has gone past the Investigational New Drug status as a treatment for OI, but it seems likely that one or more of them will in the near future.

Babies with severe OI—so fragile that they must be carried on pillows to prevent frequent breakage—are sometimes treated with splints or casts to get them through their first months safely. Somewhat older youngsters, as they reach the age to walk, can benefit from rodding, which involves inserting internal stainless steel splints in one or more long bones while the skeletal bones are still relatively soft and malleable. The rods prevent the bones from becoming deformed and also add structural strength. Rodding is usually reserved for the leg bones—the thigh and shin, though the upper and lower segments of the arm are sometimes done as well. External lightweight plastic braces are used in conjunction with rodding to secure the limb while it is healing.

With continuing research in osteogenesis imperfecta, particularly in the area of genetic screening and intervention, it seems possible that new knowledge will eventually lead to the prevention of a significant proportion of cases. For the remainder, drug treatments combined with surgery will almost surely advance, making the disorder less disabling.

Chapter Five

"SIXTY-FIVE ROSES"

CYSTIC FIBROSIS AND
OTHER METABOLIC DISORDERS

Every year about 1,000 new cases of cystic fibrosis (CF) are diagnosed in young Americans, and altogether there are perhaps 30,000 currently living with the disease in the United States. Given the frequency with which CF occurs, you might expect to find many more than that in the population, but it is a tragic fact that most people with CF die at a relatively young age. Advances in therapy over the past few years have brightened the outlook somewhat, so more than half of those afflicted with CF now survive into their late twenties and beyond. But to date, science has not succeeded in correcting the disorder of body chemicals—the failure of production of an essential metabolic protein—that lies at the root of the condition.

Cystic fibrosis, its name sometimes garbled as "sixty-five roses" by sufferers too young to pronounce it correctly, is a congenital disease that usually makes itself known symptomatically in early childhood. CF primarily afflicts people of northern European heritage. As it is a recessive condition, caused by a mutation in a single gene, it strikes only those individuals who have received defective copies of the gene from both parents. It occurs with a frequency of 1 in 2,500 births. (Black Americans, by contrast, have a 1 in 17,000 frequency of CF.)

The primary site of CF activity is in the glands that secrete mucus, sweat, and digestive enzymes to serve various functions in the body. The disorder's name refers to the particular behavior of the glands in the pancreas, the large and important organ that lies in close proximity to the stomach; they become enlarged and cystlike, eventually forming fibrous scar tissue. The mucus that originates here tends to be abnormally thick and sticky due to the lack of a special protein required for normal movement of salt into and out of cells lining the lungs and other organs. This has a cascading effect on a number of body processes. One result is that the ducts become blocked, preventing the release of critical digestive enzymes to the intestines. Much of the food that a person with CF eats consequently passes through the body essentially undigested, leaving him or her ravenously hungry and chronically undernourished and underweight.

Over time the sticky mucus also creates chronic obstructions in the body's breathing passages. Under normal circumstances our airways are bathed in a thin layer of mucus that traps inhaled particles and bacteria; like a moving conveyor belt, tiny hairs, or cilia, lining the passages normally keep the mucus flowing toward the throat, mouth, and nose where it is removed through swallowing, sneezing, coughing, and the like. But in the case of CF, the mucus overwhelms the tiny hairs of the lining and remains in place unless forcibly

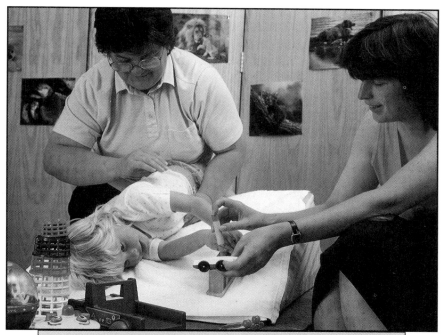

A physical therapist performs postural drainage (also known as percussion treatment) to clear the airways of a three-year-old child with cystic fibrosis.

shaken loose. With bacteria and other materials gathering undisturbed in the mucus, breathing passages become a perfect breeding ground for recurring respiratory infections. Over time the infections cause irreversible harm to branching tubes and lung tissue. Lung collapse, which is caused by the inability of the lungs to inflate due to accumulated mucus, is always a threat.

Sweat, the other secretion involved, also becomes abnormally salty, because the ducts of the sweat glands are unable to reabsorb salt, so most of it ends up leaving the body as part of sweat. Children with CF consequently release salt at about five times normal concentrations. Not only do they have unusually salty skin, but they are also very susceptible to dehydration and heat exhaustion in hot weather. (An old Scandinavian adage, dating back centuries before CF was understood, may well anticipate this fact in declaring, "Woe to the child who tastes salty when kissed, for he is bewitched and soon must die.") And in truth, the outlook until very recently was for an early death, if not in adolescence then soon after.

FINDING THE CULPRIT

The disorder was first recognized as a singular condition and given its name in 1938, when Dr. Dorothy H. Andersen, a pediatric pathologist at Columbia-Presbyterian's Babies Hospital, carried out a series of autopsies on children and infants who had died of similar symptoms. Andersen was able to confirm that all of them had damaged lungs, heart, and pancreatic tissue. As research continued, other medical scientists undertook a study of family histories and deduced the recessive inheritance pattern that underlies CF. They also zeroed in on the salt connection, from which they were able to develop the sweat test that remains one of the basic diagnostic tools.

Thanks to the ability to diagnose CF earlier in life today, children who need treatment get help sooner, preventing or slowing many of the more damaging effects of CF. To begin with, the digestive problems that go with CF can now be managed with an enriched diet and supplements taken with each meal to substitute for the missing digestive enzymes. The lost salt can be replaced, too. Parents also learn how to help reduce breathing obstructions through administering a vigorous kind of physical therapy called postural drainage. In this therapy, the youngster assumes a number of positions, including upside down, while the parent pummels and kneads the back and chest with cupped hands to literally shake the mucus loose from lungs and airways. For some youngsters this time-consuming and physically exhausting exercise needs to be done several times a day.

New drug therapies have also been devised. In 1993 a mucus-thinning (mucolytic) drug called Pulmozyme was invented by Genentech, one of the leaders in genetically engineered drugs. Heralded by the FDA as the first new product in thirty years specifically developed to treat CF, Pulmozyme is dispensed with a nebulizer, a device that reduces the liquid medication to a very fine breathable spray that is delivered deep into the lungs. According to the manufacturers, the drug works like "molecular scissors," cutting up and liquifying the secretions to keep passages open and make breathing easier. As daily doses of Pulmozyme are costly—adding up to roughly $10,000 annually for this one drug alone—Genentech established an endowment fund to help uninsured and underinsured patients obtain the drug.

In 1995, thanks to a four-year study supported by the Cystic Fibrosis Foundation, high doses of the over-the-counter drug ibuprofen, were found to reduce the rate of lung inflammation, another serious side effect of CF. And in 1997 the FDA gave orphan drug fast-track approval to the drug TOBI, an aerosolized form of the antibiotic tobramycin used in combating chronic lung infection. For some time TOBI had been administered intravenously when CF youngsters were so sick as to need hospitalization, but under the new arrangements they could take it at home, before their condition worsened. And this was important because it meant that patients could nip potentially serious infections early and without disrupting their lives.

RADICAL STRATEGIES

Surgical transplantation is another new avenue of treatment in some advanced cases. In January 2000, nineteen-year-old Darrell Hedgecoth of Ashland City, Tennessee, became one of a handful of people to receive a triple transplant—heart, lungs, and liver—to save his life.[1] Hedgecoth, who had been diagnosed with CF at three months of age, had seen his health gradually deteriorate over his first twelve years, until his lungs had become so scarred and damaged that he had to limit activities. In high school he had to be home schooled, and six months before being placed on a transplant waiting list in July 1999, he had been tethered to an oxygen tank twenty-four hours a day. This severely limited his ability to enjoy even the simplest pleasures, but Darrell was blessed with a naturally optimistic spirit, and he continued to hope that some miracle would come along. Each day that he lived while waiting seemed an added gift.

At dawn on a late January morning Darrell received the long-awaited phone call telling him that a near-perfect match had become available as the result of a fatal motorcycle accident. Hedgecoth and his family rushed to Vanderbilt Hospital in Nashville where the transplant team was standing by. The surgery went smoothly, and six hours after it was over, the boy was breathing well. Within a dozen days he was able to go home. Since that time, Darrell has been able to resume a near normal life and to think about the future, something that had for so long seemed beyond his wildest dreams.

But the really big news in CF has been triggered by the discovery of the defective gene responsible for CF. The basic science was completed in 1989 when a large group of medical collaborators, led by Canadians Lap-Chee Tsui and John Riordan of the Hospital for Sick Children in Toronto, and by Francis S. Collins, then of the University of Michigan, announced that it had isolated the target gene on Chromosome 7.[2] (Collins would go on to lead the government/academic team that deciphered the human genome in 2001.) The CF researchers went on to note that the gene normally gives rise to a protein that they called "cystic fibrosis transmembrane conductance regulator" (CFTR) on account of its influence over the movement of sodium and chloride into and out of cells. This initial finding gave hope that the defect responsible for CF might ultimately be correctable through the insertion of a "good" gene in place of the "bad" gene.

As it turns out, the problem is still more complicated. The researchers had initially thought that the CF mutation was always the same, but they have since realized that though perhaps 70 percent of cystic fibrosis patients share the same mutation, another 30 percent have any one of a hundred or more other equally small mutations. This distinction probably accounts for the distinctive disease spectrum associated with CF: why some individuals have more devastating CF than others. Those who inherit two identical copies of the mutation get a double dose of serious symptoms while those who inherit differently skewed CF genes are less incapacitated.

Despite this added wrinkle, researchers continue to believe that they will someday find a reliable way to repair the deviant gene by inserting the correct amino acid where it is needed. One route under study is to modify a common cold virus to act as the vector, or delivery vehicle. Viruses by their nature must invade cells in order to complete their life cycle and multiply. Cold viruses are specifically programmed to target cells lining the respiratory tract, so they would seem to be perfect vectors. The idea then is to insert the desired genes into a colony of deactivated cold virus vectors, encourage them to infect the same mucus cells where CFTR genes are primarily expressed, and hope that the viruses will step aside and allow the new genes to function normally. Another possible approach is to develop a synthetic vector—unlike cold or any other existing viruses but of proven safety. The third approach is to create some other nonviral means of entry such as a liposome or fat capsule capable of insinuating itself into the gene. So far, the work is proceeding slowly and with mixed results, and no one can safely predict when any of these techniques will become viable treatments for CF.

Financial assistance in these pursuits comes in part from governmental agencies like the NIH. But major funding—$130 million this year alone—is also supplied by the Cystic Fibrosis Foundation, which was established in 1955 to focus attention on this life-shortening genetic disease. The foundation, which was the first privately run health agency in the United States to create its own network of research centers, supports major programs at a number of universities and medical schools. It is also working on the front lines, promoting CF drug development with more than twenty new drugs currently in various stages of clinical testing. And to help patients and researchers alike, it works to link patients to clinical drug trials. Lastly, the Cystic

Fibrosis Foundation supports 115 CF-dedicated centers nationwide, some within major community hospitals, others at major teaching hospitals, but all provide comprehensive diagnosis and treatment and counseling to patients and their families.[3]

TAY-SACHS DISEASE

As orphan diseases go, CF is one of the more widespread metabolic disorders in the U.S. population. (Diabetes is *the* most common and is not considered an "orphan" by any standards.) But there are many other orphan diseases in this category that affect truly small populations. Often these rare conditions are associated with groups of people who have historically lived in isolated communities where there was little opportunity or desire to intermarry with people of other cultures. One particularly striking example is Tay-Sachs disease (TSD), which primarily strikes the offspring of Ashkenazi Jews, though it is also found infrequently in French Canadians of the St. Lawrence region, certain Cajun clusters in Louisiana, and in some Amish communities. How the Ashkenazis in particular have come to be so closely associated with Tay-Sachs, and how they have chosen to address their predisposition to this genetic condition, is a fascinating story in itself.

TSD is an autosomal recessive disorder, meaning that it is passed on by two "carrier" parents. It was first described in the 1880s by a British ophthalmologist, Warren Tay, and a New York City neurologist, Bernard Sachs. Each man had many immigrant Ashkenazi Jews among his patients and was drawn to learn more about this rare affliction. Though neither Dr. Tay nor Dr. Sachs could know it at the time, we now can say that affected babies have inherited two defective copies (i.e., one from each parent) of the gene responsible for producing the enzyme hexosaminidase A, whose role in the body is to break down or metabolize fatty substances. The carrier parents are healthy because they have one dominant normal gene that masks the recessive defective gene. They are thus able to produce half the normal amount of hex-A, as it is familiarly known, which is enough of the enzyme to carry out essential metabolic function. Consequently, they experience no adverse health effects. But when two such carriers conceive as a couple, they have a one-in-four chance of producing a child who has no gene for hex-A at all. This unfortunate child will not be able to metabolize fatty substances; rather, fatty substances will build up to toxic levels, particularly around cells of the brain and nervous system, causing normal neurological functions to become increasingly more difficult.

The newborn with TSD usually appears healthy at birth but within the first year of life, as the stored material accumulates, muscle development slows and then reverses. These so-called floppy babies have difficulty rolling over, crawling, feeding, and swallowing. Seizures occur, and the infant shows general unresponsiveness except to sound or bright light, where the response may be excessive (startle response). A characteristic marker that is visible upon medical examination is a tiny cherry-red spot in the retina of the eye. As symptoms worsen, mental retardation sets in, the child loses sight, and eventually he or she becomes paralyzed and unresponsive to any stimulation. No treatment exists for TSD, and the condition is fatal in all cases, usually between the third and fifth years of life.

The Ashkenazi Jews' vulnerability is thought to have been introduced into their gene pool sometime after the Second Diaspora in A.D. 70, when thousands of Jews were driven out of the Holy Land to scatter across the known world. The Ashkenazis went first to parts of what would later be called Germany and subsequently to Russia and Poland. It is thought that the single cell mutation occurred sometime after their resettlement in eastern Europe.

Because the ultraorthodox Ashkenazis married exclusively within their culture, sometimes practicing polygamy, it developed over time that the mutation was passed on over and over to ever widening circles but only within their closed community. (One scientist has advanced the intriguing hypothesis that while infants who have TSD may die of the disorder, carriers may somehow benefit from the single defective gene by being more tolerant to tuberculosis (TB) than noncarriers. As generations of eastern European Jews were forced to live in urban ghettos where conditions leading to TB posed an even greater threat to the group's survival, there may have been some selective advantage. If so, this would be a relationship of genetic mutation to an environmental stress, not unlike that of sickle cell anemia and malaria among people of African and Mediterranean ancestries.)

Whatever the explanation, other populations in eastern Europe who presumably followed other faiths and who tended to live less urban lives remained virtually untouched. It is estimated today that one in every thirty people of Ashkenazi Jewish heritage is a carrier. Carriers, as we have seen, do not "have" the disease and show no outward evidence that they carry the gene, but they are capable of passing TSD along to their children if the other parent is also a carrier. (As this is an autosomal recessive genetic disorder, such parents have a one-in-four chance with each pregnancy that the child will be affected.) Because members of orthodox com-

91

munities of Ashkenazi descent continue to marry and procreate almost exclusively among their own narrowly defined group, the Ashkenazis are theoretically as vulnerable as ever. Indeed, this is true even in the United States, which has a sizable population of eastern European Jews, particularly living in and around many urban centers.

Back in 1969, John O'Brien, MD, a professor of neurosciences at the University of California, isolated the genetic defect causing TSD.[4] Once the relationship between the defective gene for hex-A and TSD was understood, it became possible to develop a biochemical test that looked for hex-A activity or lack of it and to identify carriers of the genetic disorder. Initially, the test was offered to parents only after they had produced an infant with TSD and wanted to test themselves for the mutation or test prenatally to know the health outlook of the next child they were carrying. As many of the people for whom such a test was relevant had firm religious objections to both contraception and abortion, the test had enjoyed only limited use. Despite the fear that parents inevitably felt, they continued to bear more children and hope for the best. But with a one-in-four chance that each infant would be born with the disease, and with orthodox Jewish families traditionally favoring large families, many couples experienced devastating losses over and over.

Rabbi Josef Ekstein, a leader within the Williamsburg community of Hassidim in Brooklyn, New York, knew the tragic consequences personally.[5] Not only did he often counsel bereaved members of the congregation, but he and his wife had watched helplessly as four of their ten children were born seemingly healthy only to become fatally stricken within months. Aware of the new screening test available, Rabbi

Ekstein began to think about ways to prevent such tragedies without stepping outside of religious doctrine. In 1983 he founded Dor Yeshorim, Hebrew for "Generation of the Righteous," a low-cost premarital genetic testing program. The program quickly gained the sponsorship of numbers of synagogues, especially in the ultraorthodox Hassidic Jewish communities around New York and Chicago, where arranged marriages are the usual practice. (Arranged marriages are based on what is considered best for the community. Matches are made by the rabbi or by a recognized *shadchen*, which means intermediary or "matchmaker," without concern for romantic attachment or even acquaintanceship on the part of those involved.)

When an unmarried Hassidic woman reaches age eighteen and a Hassidic man age twenty, they are given a blood test that screens for TSD. The lab handling the tests assigns a code number to each sample and the results are stored anonymously in a database accessible only to rabbis and matchmakers. Preparatory to finalizing a match, the intermediary submits the code numbers of the prospective bride and groom to find out if the match is "good" or not. If the laboratory comes back with a negative finding, meaning that each of the people is a carrier, the match is cancelled and another one investigated without the individuals ever learning their status. Implicit in this process is avoiding the effects of genetic stigmatization.

In the case of couples who do not use the services of a matchmaker, the procedure is somewhat the same: If only one of the pair is a carrier of the TSD mutation, and the results thus favor healthy offspring, no information beyond that fact is given to anyone. Only when both individuals are carriers are they told, at which point they must decide whether to go forward with their marriage or not. Apparently very few do. According to Jayn Gershkowitz, executive director of the National Tay-Sachs and Allied Diseases Association in Boston, the screening and educational programs widely used among the Ashkenazi population in the United States and Canada have led to a 95 percent reduction in TSD births since the early 1970s.[6]

Chapter Six

THE TROUBLED BRAIN

OBSESSIVE-COMPULSIVE AND OTHER MOOD DISORDERS

Dr. Samuel Johnson, eighteenth-century English lexicographer, poet, playwright, and critic, is regarded as one of the wisest and most talented men of his age, or of any age for that matter. Yet Dr. Johnson had some seemingly odd habits. For one thing, he found it virtually impossible to enter or leave a doorway without going through a series of elaborate gyrations and gestures. His great admirer, James Boswell, records that Johnson had a "peculiarity, of which none of his friends even ventured to ask an explanation. . . . This was his anxious care to go out or in at a door or passage, by a certain number of steps from a certain point, or at least so as that either his right or his left foot (I am not certain which), should constantly make the first actual movement when he came close."[1] Others noted that Johnson invariably touched every post as he walked along the street, retracing steps if he missed one, that he set his feet carefully to avoid ever stepping on cracks in the pavement, and "would give a sudden spring and make such an extensive stride over the threshold, as if he were trying for a wager how far he could stride."[2] Fortunate to live in a more forgiving and slow-paced era, Johnson was regarded by his friends as demonstrating nothing more than the eccentricities of a great mind.

Modern psychiatrists and neurologists, those specialists in the workings of the brain, know otherwise. They recognize in Johnson's behavior one of the classic rituals of someone with obsessive-compulsive disorder (OCD). OCD is a brain disease. NORD estimates that there may be as many as five million Americans, or 2 percent to 3 percent of the population, with the condition, but that it varies widely in severity so that only a fraction are impaired enough to need treatment. The typical age of onset for boys is six to fifteen, for girls considerably later, in the years between twenty and thirty.

OCD tends to run in families. A person with OCD has a 25 percent chance of having a blood relative who has it. Among identical twins, the likelihood is substantially higher still. To date, the disorder's underlying cause or causes have not been identified, but the prevalent theory is that this is a complex disease involving multiple genes. As each of the multiple genes is thought to send out a weak signal—unlike one of the simpler one-gene "Mendelian disorders" such as CF—it is as difficult to detect as a proverbial needle in a haystack.

Making the task of studying this disorder still more difficult is the fact that researchers typically rely on clusters of subjects within a reasonable geographic area to carry out their studies, and clusters of OCD patients are hard to come by. Lastly, OCD seems to need an environmental stressor to be expressed: triggers may include physical abuse; sharp changes in living, school, or working situations; or an emotional loss such as the death of a parent. A severe childhood illness might also be a trigger. A group of researchers at the NIMH have suggested that a streptococcus bacteria—the sort that causes strep throat and rheumatic fever—may play a role in triggering some cases of OCD. They note that MRI brain scans of some OCD patients who have had such infections show slight enlargement in the basal ganglia areas of the brain, and that metabolic activity there is abnormally fast; this suggests that some chemical or biological aspect of mental processing may have been altered. Serotonin, a chemical that plays an essential role in transmitting nerve impulses or messages from one nerve cell to another, may be the culprit; tests indicate that OCD sufferers have less serotonin available than the rest of us, so the nervous system must struggle harder to communicate.

The obsession component of OCD usually centers around undesirable, recurrent, and disturbing thoughts, mental images, or impulses that regularly force themselves to the front of the mind; this produces severe anxiety and feelings of dread, fright, disgust, or apprehension. The compulsions—repetitive or ritualized behaviors—are performed uncontrollably in an effort to address and control the obsessions, and because they usually bring temporary relief, doing them reinforces the desire to do them again.

In the most common pairing of cause and effect seen among OCD patients, it's a fear of filth or contamination that prompts the person to wash his or her hands over and over every day or to clean floors, walls, and countertops interminably. Disturbing thoughts of being harmed may lead to repetitive "checking," the second most common behavior; the worried or anxious person ritually checks security locks on doors and windows, or the controls on the kitchen stove out of fear of fire, not just once or twice but ten, twenty, one hundred times a day. On each occasion the worry turns out to be false. Still other less frequent OCD behaviors are ordering and arranging items, touching parts of the body, hoarding objects, exaggerated list making, repeating words, repeating gestures or movements, and counting. People with OCD are typically very aware that they are behaving in abnormal ways and desperately want to stop, but they can't. Some have compared the affliction to having a bad case of hiccups that won't go away.

One of the problems in diagnosing OCD is that many if not most of us display a few of these symptoms now and then. But the occasional "quirks" ordinary folks have are nothing more than common nervous "tics," superstitions, or habits; they are neither so important nor so frequent as to interfere with our lives. Unlike people with genuine OCD, most of us grow out of our nervous habits eventually or are able to stop on our own if sufficiently bothered by them.

Another complicating factor in diagnosis is that other conditions bear striking similarities and may respond to some of the same treatments. For example, some movement or tic disorders—particularly Tourette syndrome with its uncontrollable snorts and shouts and utterances of inappropriate words (obscenities and the like)—may sometimes be mistaken for OCD. Research has shown, in fact, that TS and OCD are statistically more likely to appear in the same families, with girls tending to have the former and boys the latter. TS may also exist as a secondary disorder in persons with full-fledged OCD. Trichotillomania—an extreme form of compulsive hair pulling that leaves the individual bald, as well as such eating disorders as anorexia nervosa (self-starvation) and bulimia (alternate binge eating and self-induced purging), panic disorders, phobias, substance abuse, and pathological gambling may briefly be confused with OCD because of their repetitive nature and the individual's inability to resist them. But in each of these cases the person with the disorder is actually deriving some pleasure, albeit a self-destructive one, from the characteristic act.

Bipolar or manic depression is another seemingly related disorder, in that both OCD and bipolar disorder are often dominated by extended periods of depression. But unlike the OCD individual who may be depressed over his or her inability to stop what he or she recognizes as a "pointless" activity, the bipolar person is caught up in his or her actions and believes them wholly justified by the circumstances. We'll talk about bipolar disorder at greater length in a later part of this chapter. Schizophrenia, still another brain disorder, often prompts a number of "compulsive" behaviors, but the actions are in response to delusions—inner voices that seem to command the actions—rather than biochemical compulsions.

Still another condition sometimes confused with OCD is obsessive-compulsive *personality* disorder (OCPD), a psychiatric condition. Individuals with the psychiatric disorder do not act in response to genuine obsessions and compulsions, but they demonstrate a rigid, inflexible need for orderliness, perfection, and control in their work, their social interactions, or any other situation. This may lead them to check things repeatedly or to repeat instructions over and over. But there is conscious intent in their action, however misguided.

Before the advent of modern drugs and behavioral therapy, there was no help for persons with OCD. Those with mild to moderate cases (performing ritual actions only occasionally or at worst doing so two or three hours of the day) suffered in silence and ignorance. They tried to disguise their activities with other gestures that they hoped would be seen as more appropriate, while going about the rest of their life as best they could. Privately, they worried about their sanity or whether they were bewitched. And if theirs was a severe form of OCD (taking up many hours in the day and tending toward extreme actions), their families often sought to hide them away in back rooms or in institutions out of "shame." In the 1930s and 1940s, psychosurgery or lobotomy was heralded as therapy in some extreme cases of OCD. A Portuguese neurosurgeon, Egas Moniz, won a Nobel Prize in medicine for developing the technique, which involved cutting away certain neural connections in the prefrontal parts of the brain. The surgery did in fact stop obsessive and compulsive actions, but in the process, patients were left virtually helpless or without abilities—such as memory and judgment—critical to function as an intelligent human being. The cure was soon understood to be worse than the disorder, and in due course it was abandoned.

A great deal has changed in recent years in the way OCD is treated. A range of medications reduces the underlying obsessions as well as the depression and stress that accompany the behaviors. Specifically, a group of antidepressants known as serotonin reuptake inhibitors (SRIs) slows the reabsorption (neutralization) of serotonin after it is emitted by a transmitting nerve cell in the process of sending a message. This makes more of the chemical messenger available where there was an insufficiency before, in effect adding "more bounce" to nerve transmission in the brain. Changes in serotonin levels also seem to alter the activity of other brain systems, though *seem* is the operative word. Researchers still don't understand all the underlying mechanisms involved.

The first SRI, clomipramine or Anafranil, was developed by Ciba-Geigy early in the 1970s; clomipramine was available in Canada, Mexico, and Europe for many years before patients could routinely obtain it in the United States, because of obstacles in the clinical testing and approval process here. Not only is Anafranil widely used now, but so are several newer drugs called selective serotonin reuptake inhibitors (SSRIs), including Luvox, Prozac, Zoloft, Paxil, and Celexa. As every patient is unique, and as the patient's age must be taken into account in prescribing, physicians often have to try several of these drugs and varied dosages to get satisfactory results.

Behavioral therapies are also used in conjunction with the drugs. This typically combines techniques called exposure and response prevention. In the exposure part, a patient who has agreed to cooperate in the treatment is deliberately exposed to feared objects or images, either directly or indirectly by triggering the imagination. When the exposure triggers the compulsion to act, the therapist discourages or prevents the usual response. A typical exposure-response prevention drill might be to force the compulsive washer to touch something believed to be fearfully contaminated, like a doorknob, and then prevent him or her from washing hands for several hours. When the treatment works well, the patient is gradually desensitized to the triggering event; upon each successive exposure he or she feels less anxiety, until it becomes possible to do without the actions at all for extended periods of time. Notably, the one therapy that seems to have little effect on reducing OCD itself is traditional psychotherapy, because the causes of the disorder are fundamentally biological rather than emotional. On the other hand, patients who have become so isolated through the years because of shame and embarrassment, may benefit from this kind of counseling simply to gain self-confidence in living normally.

BIPOLAR DISORDER

Bipolar disorder, more commonly known as manic depression, is a mental disorder in which intense mood swings occur. The term *bipolar* refers to the fact that persons suffering from the disorder go from one "pole," or extreme, to the other in behavior. When they are in the manic phase, they feel expansive, euphoric, irrationally optimistic, extremely sociable, generous, invincible. They lose rational judgment and their self-esteem soars. In particularly extreme cases, a person in the manic phase develops illusions of grandeur, imagining himself or herself to be someone of great importance, such as the president of the United States, the pope, or even God. While on this "high" they may call people on the phone at all hours of the day or night; have difficulty sleeping; become easily distracted; and often carry out actions as though there were no consequences, such as running up charges on credit cards and/or participating in dangerous activities. They may dress in bizarre ways, give away their possessions, talk compulsively to strangers. They may be irritable if others are unwilling to support them in their manic behaviors. Their speech is often inflated and they talk louder, faster, often theatrically. Sometimes a "flight of ideas"—one patient has described them as "like shooting stars"—bombards their mind so that their ability to process words and sentences is impaired; everything comes out in an incomprehensible jumble, of which they are unaware.

When later these individuals descend into the depressive phase of their mental disorder, they become anxious, tearful, sad, physically tired, and inclined to sleep for long periods; often they are overwhelmed with feelings of worthlessness and guilt, brought on in part by a belated awareness of their manic behavior. They may withdraw from friends and family and become incapable of taking any positive actions on their own behalf. They may neglect to eat, to wash, or to change their clothes for days or even weeks. Some manic-depressives become obsessed with their health or full of phobias that resemble those of OCD. Some experience bouts of depression so deep that they cannot imagine any reason for living and attempt suicide. Others become angry and hostile when others try to help them. And their speech, if they speak at all, may be monotone and slow, as though even this effort is more than they can handle.

Manic depression bears some gross similarities to other forms of mental illness, but its specific combination of factors ultimately distinguishes it from the rest. Some of the look-alikes are clinical or major depression, which does not alternate with manic phases; and seasonal affective disorder (SAD), which is a form of seasonal mild depression associated with insufficient production of certain hormones that depend on sunlight for their manufacture. Anxiety disorders, including post-traumatic stress disorder and OCD, can appear along with manic depression in some cases, too.

The episodic cycles of the disorder vary widely. Some individuals go from mania to depression and back in rapid shifts, so that both extremes are seen in a single day. Some have long periods of depression followed very infrequently by brief bouts of mania; some enjoy months and years of normal functioning only to have some unknown event trigger a bipolar episode; still others find the episodes growing in frequency and severity as they age.

Classic bipolar manic depression is traceable to the genes, but precisely which one or ones is as yet undetermined. In 1987 a group of scientists announced what they thought was a thrilling discovery: They had succeeded in locating a gene for manic depression in a large Amish family living in Lancaster, Pennsylvania.[3] They said the gene was located near the tip of the short arm of Chromosome 11, one of the 23 pairs of chromosomes that make up the human genetic code. Had they been right, this would have been the very first proof of a psychiatric disorder being traceable to a specific genetic mutation. But in due course the researchers had to retract their claim. New information from other members of the same Amish clan, and from other researchers who had equally persuasive evidence for other chromosomal locations, has cast doubt on the accuracy or interpretations of the earlier studies.

Nowadays, the best thinking is that manic depression, like OCD, schizophrenia, and a good number of other complex disorders, is oligogenic. That is, these disorders occur only when several genes somehow misfire and when they are further pushed to action by some external (environmental) trigger. Bipolar disorder does tend to run in families, so a significant proportion of the genes involved are thought to be inherited. Developments in brain imaging technology (especially

104

PET scans, which permit researchers to view moving pictures of the chemical and biological activity of the brain as they are happening in a given patient) will almost certainly add important additional information to what is now known.

According to projections compiled by the NIMH, more than two million American adults, or about 1 percent of the population age eighteen and older, have bipolar manic depression in any given year. Fortunately, only a small portion of these have symptoms severe enough to interfere with daily function, while many more find the disorder a periodic burden to their enjoyment of life. The disorder typically develops in late adolescence or early adulthood, though it occasionally has its onset earlier and may, in some instances, not make an appearance until relatively late in life. It also appears to affect more females than males. Once it appears, it must be regarded as a lifelong illness capable of returning even after long periods of quiescence.

Without knowledge of the multiple genes involved in manic depression, its precise cause cannot be identified except to say that it is a disorder of brain chemicals. In all likelihood, some chemical interference in the activity of the neurotransmitters serotonin, norepinephrine, and dopamine are involved. And it is this interruption that somehow causes messages to go "haywire," causing the extreme mood swings.

Standard treatment of manic depression these days is typically managed by a psychiatrist, a medical doctor with expertise in the diagnosis and treatment of mental diseases. Treatment is based primarily on the use of medications known as mood stabilizers with additional support through various "talking" psychosocial therapies in which the therapist, the patient, and sometimes other family members participate on a regular basis.

Lithium, the first of a long line of these mood-stabilizing psychotropic drugs, was introduced in 1949. A chance discovery by Dr. John Cade, an Australian physician at a psychiatric hospital in Melbourne, provided the first real indication that moods had a chemical basis.[4] Cade discovered lithium's value while conducting experiments on laboratory guinea pigs. Injections of lithium carbonate made the guinea pigs unusually placid. Not restricted by the kinds of rules that are in place today, the doctor went on to give a similar injection to one of his depressed patients, a fifty-one-year-old man who had been in mental institutions for twenty years. In just five days, the patient went from being incoherent, dirty, and destructive to exhibiting remarkable calm; he cleaned his room, attended to his person, and began to carry on normal conversations. Two months later, with repeated doses of lithium carbonate, Cade's patient was able to leave the hospital and go home to his family.

Lithium for depression led researchers to try it for the extreme highs of mania, and once again, the drug has proved remarkably effective in most cases. SSRIs like Prozac, tricyclic antidepressants, and anticonvulsants are also helpful for some patients. Therapeutic practice these days is to maintain patients on a continuous drug regimen even during periods of relatively normal mood levels. This often reduces the frequency and duration of cycles, allowing a substantial percentage of patients to lead normal, even highly successful lives. Almost certainly, more drugs will be developed when the genetic sites involved in manic depression have been isolated and pharmaceutical researchers know the truly narrow targets at which they aim.

In the rare cases that have proved unresponsive to standard drug and psychosocial treatments, electrocon-

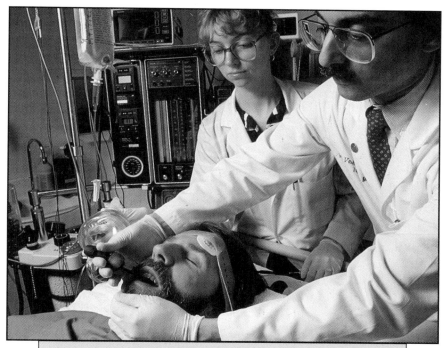

Electroconvulsive therapy requires careful preparation of the patient by the doctor and anesthesiologist. The doctor is inserting a mouthpiece designed to prevent injury during a brain seizure.

vulsive therapy (ECT) or "shock" treatment is sometimes applied. Shock treatments were first used to treat mental disorders by Giovanni Aldini, an eighteenth-century physicist who experimented at length with the effects of electricity on the body, using himself as guinea pig.[5] Aldini found that by putting electrodes in both ears, or in one ear and in his mouth, or in his nose and on his forehead, he could elicit some very "disagreeable" sensations, including convulsions, but he thought they might serve as a means of "rearranging the functions of the brain" in conditions of "melancholy" or depression.

Others continued his work intermittently, and in 1938, shock therapy was formally introduced as a recognized therapy for depression and schizophrenia. Nowadays, patients are given anesthesia and muscle relaxants to prevent any pain or damage from the muscle spasms that the resulting seizures induce. Two padded electrodes are then placed on the temples, and a controlled electric pulse is delivered to the electrodes to cause a brain seizure. The seizure evidently causes brain chemicals to be released, and this usually brings improved mood, if not immediately, then after three or more treatments. The patient awakes feeling mildly discomfited and with little or no memory of the event.

Herbal supplements have also been tried in the treatment of manic depression, with St. John's wort (*Hypericum perforatum*) the leading choice. While there is some anecdotal indication that it may relieve very mild unipolar depression in some patients, there is no evidence at all that it can help bipolar disorder. And it may, in fact, provide a barrier to the most effective use of some recognized drugs.

Chapter Seven

THE BOY IN THE BUBBLE

SCID AND OTHER IMMUNODEFICIENCY DISORDERS

When Carol Ann and David Vetter Jr. had their first son, they did what many proud new parents do: they named him after the father. But within six months, baby David was dead, the victim of a very rare disorder known as severe combined immune deficiency (SCID).[1] Specialists at Baylor College of Medicine in Houston, Texas, near where the family lived, told the grieving parents that their child had been born with an error in his thymus. (The thymus is a ductless organ belonging to the lymphatic system. It's found in the lower part of the neck and it's crucial in the first years of life to developing immunity to the myriad agents that attack the body.) Though the Vetters' baby had enjoyed some disease resistance immediately after birth because he still carried his mother's antibodies, he had gradually weakened with each passing week as his own system took over and his thymus failed to do its job. Every passing germ caused mild fevers, skin rashes, or stomach disorders. Eventually, not even the wearing of masks and gloves on the part of his caregivers or the disinfecting of the room in which he slept were enough to protect little David. In the end it was probably some common infectious agent that killed him, something that almost any other baby would have tossed off with ease.

This being the 1970s, when relatively little was understood about the genetics of SCID or most other birth defects, the doctors pondering baby David's disorder thought his lack of adequate immunity was probably the result of a random genetic mutation. If this were so, the chance of it happening to the Vetters a second time would be extremely rare, perhaps one in ten thousand. On the other hand, they counseled that in the unlikely event that the genetic defect was carried on the mother's chromosomes, there was a fifty-fifty risk of recurrence. But even then, the doctors were optimistic. With medicine making such remarkable strides, they predicted that a cure might lie just over the horizon. By taking proper precautions from the moment of delivery, they forecast, a SCID child could be isolated and kept safe from external infection until a way was found to give him a new and self-sustaining immune system.

Indeed, one of the doctors on the team had previously been a participant in the care of a set of French twins under somewhat similar circumstances. The twins had been treated in a sterile environment until, at age three, their immune systems had developed to a point where the twins could be safely introduced to the world at large. Meanwhile, because medical research groups within the American government were intensely interested in learning more about immunological disorders, the NIH was offering to underwrite the extraordinary costs of caring for the next Vetter child if indeed he or she had SCID. In return, the NIH and other researchers would have full access to medical data useful to their studies.

Under the circumstances, the Vetters decided to have another child, and on September 21, 1971, the baby was delivered by caesarian section at St. Luke's Episcopal Hospital in Houston, Texas. For the second time it was a boy, and for the second time the parents named him David. In the moments immediately after delivery, the doctors could not know for sure what might lie ahead, but they acted with maximum caution. The newborn was immediately placed in a prearranged sterile plastic isolation capsule and hurried over to the adjoining Texas Children's Hospital for observation. The bad news was not long in coming, however. This David, like his predecessor, was a SCID baby.

The Vetters were told that their baby would have to stay in the hospital indefinitely, where he would be kept safe in his plastic safety bubble until some means of providing him with a functioning immune system could be devised. Until such time, they could only touch him, feed him, care for him, and play with him through gloved portals in the side of an air-supported but otherwise sealed container.

Sadly, David lived that way for the next twelve years. As he grew and became more active, he was transferred to ever larger "bubbles," and on rare occasions to a temporary "space suit." But whatever the containment facility, David's protective personal space was always physically awkward, limiting, and noisy, the result of the ventilation system that kept the bubble inflated and David breathing twenty-four hours a day. Under special circumstances, David, along with his

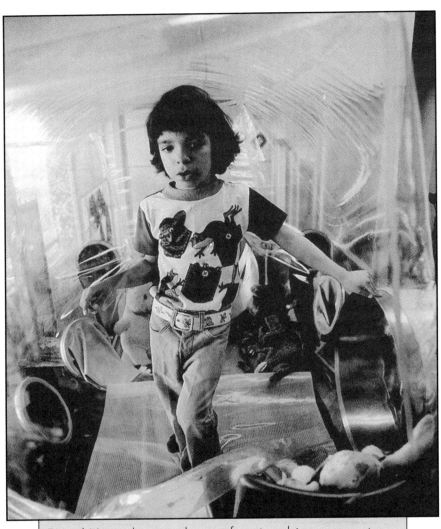

David Vetter, born without a functional immune system, spent all of his twelve years of life in a protective "bubble" environment. Here, five-year-old David romps in his very limited world in a Houston, Texas hospital.

"bubble" and various professional caregivers, could be transported to his parents' home for visits, but he was sentenced to remain essentially alone for his own survival. He would never know his parents' touch, would never play with other children, would never breathe "fresh air" or wander outdoors. He would never even be allowed to eat unsterilized food or explore the delights of ordinary toys, books, clothing, or any other item that had not been sanitized and purified first.

By any measure it was not much of a life, but David's situation fascinated others and he became an unwilling celebrity. Magazines wrote stories about him. Feature movies were made about him. Medical researchers came to observe and take notes. Engineers and technologists devoted their spare time to devising better equipment to make his life more comfortable. And a parade of official visitors stopped by to view his odd circumstances, as though he were a circus attraction. No child before him had ever been raised in this manner, and everyone speculated as to the effect it was having on his psychological well-being. As it became increasingly clear that a "cure" was still years away and that David might be facing "imprisonment" for the rest of his life, the moral dilemma of maintaining him in this horrible existence became more apparent. Ethicists, physicians, journalists, theologians, psychologists, and ordinary citizens took sides in a continuing debate over what to do with "the boy in the bubble." Even David, who was highly intelligent despite his limited experience of the "real world," came to believe that he would rather be dead than go on as he was. There were no easy answers.

Eventually, David's doctors proposed the only solution they had, explaining that at best it was highly risky: They would transplant healthy but imperfectly matched human bone marrow cells from a sibling into David's system with the hope that the cells would multiply and eventually give him the natural immunity he lacked. David's parents, who had lived these years watching David suffer, decided to take the chance. David, who had grown increasingly angry and moody, said he had no faith in the effort and just wished for the whole thing to be over.

On October 21, 1983, a month after his twelfth birthday, marrow was drawn from one of David's sisters and dripped slowly into David's bloodstream. At first the transplant seemed to be successful. (Outright rejection, which is usually the largest hurdle in transplantations, does not occur in SCID, because there is no immune system to recognize and reject foreign antibodies.) The doctors cautiously dared to think that David might soon be able to leave his bubble and live a normal life for the first time. But within six weeks, problems began to surface. By February, David was very sick with multiple infections for which no medications were adequate. The transplanted cells had not prospered as hoped.

Despite intensive efforts to save him, young David died on February 22, 1984. An autopsy later revealed that despite his sister's being prescreened for anything that might be toxic to David, her donated marrow had contained undetected amounts of the common Epstein-Barr virus. Because David's immune response was abnormal, the virus had flourished and had eventually produced Burkitt's lymphoma, a cancerous condition easily capable of killing him.

SCID TODAY

In the nearly twenty years that have passed since David Vetter's death, notable progress has been made in understanding the incidence, origins, and behavior of

SCID. Modern medicine has also made remarkable strides in treating SCID, so much so that they can now intervene in ways that allow many SCID individuals to live a normal life. But more of that later.

We now know that there are some seventy kinds of *primary* immune deficiency diseases.[2] This is in distinction to *secondary* immune deficiencies that evolve as the result of some other primary triggering event: AIDS, various kinds of leukemia, and prolonged regimens of radiation and/or chemotherapy can all cause secondary immune deficiencies. Each of the primary immune deficiency diseases is derived from the failure of some specific gene to produce an enzyme essential to the chemical workings of the immune system. We also know that SCID is exceedingly rare, with an incidence of something like 1 in 100,000 if we combine all kinds, and more like 1 in a million for some variants. This extreme rarity matters because the research, treatments, and drugs needed are often different for each kind, but the effort that must go into finding solutions is often as great as that required for a major disease.

The symptoms of SCID are now better understood, too. Symptoms usually begin to appear shortly after birth as the immunity derived from the mother begins to wear off. Even in the absence of direct contact with a disease carrier, and despite the parents' best efforts to protect their newborn, common bacterial, viral, and fungal infections can erupt, any one of them the result of opportunistic organisms that literally surround us, waiting for the opportunity to hit a vulnerable target. SCID babies also tend to suffer serious consequences from the ordinary immunizations routinely given in the first months of life; in these immunodeficient children even the most attenuated vaccines have the capacity to flower into the disease they are meant to protect against. We also know that all forms of SCID are heri-

115

table, either as a recessive or an X-linked disorder. (The gene for David Vetter's SCID was identified in 1993 as a defect in the gene involved in bringing T cells to maturity; this particular error is thought to be X-linked and consequently carried by males and females but usually expressed only in male offspring. Other forms of SCID are present equally in both sexes.)

When SCID is suspected, closer physical examination of the youngster usually reveals that the thymus is underdeveloped; similarly, the tonsils and adenoids, two other players in the lymphatic system, may be smaller than normal. Another indicator is found in a blood smear test. Under the microscope, the blood of SCID individuals usually has severely reduced counts of two varieties of specialized white cells involved in cellular immune response. One group is the B lymphocytes, which generates the antibodies that disarm antigens on the surface of invading microorganisms. The other set is the so-called killer T lymphocytes, which launches a kind of chemical warfare against foreign or abnormal cells.

It is also possible these days to diagnose some forms of SCID before birth (in utero). This is done by a procedure known as amniocentesis. A needle is inserted through the mother's abdomen until the tip reaches the amniotic fluid that surrounds the fetus, and a small sample is drawn. The fluid, which contains dilute concentrations of the substances, including chromosomes, found in the fetus's blood, is then studied for specific abnormalities. Arriving in this life with SCID, however, is no longer necessarily a death sentence. As Dr. Rebecca Buckley, chief of Duke University Medical School's division of pediatric immunology, says, "Every baby with SCID could be cured today if diagnosed early enough. Rather, SCID should be considered a pediatric emergency."[3]

At Duke and at other specialized children's hospitals, emergency treatment for these children centers around the early use of several remarkable new drugs, some of which have been developed under the orphan drug program. Most notably, the orphan drug Adagen was approved in 1990; a long-term course of therapy involving weekly injections of Adagen, which replaces a key enzyme that is lacking, can actually restore the immune function of some SCID children to near normal. Several antibiotics have also been developed to treat a rare and particularly hardy form of bacterial pneumonia that targets SCID children. Bone marrow transplants, such as that used in David Vetter's case, continue to be highly risky, but there are dozens of survivor children around these days to prove that it can be done successfully. Nowadays, more sophisticated methods of screening donor marrow are employed, and patients are prepared for bone marrow transplants with doses of chemotherapy and radiation therapy to further enhance their body's ability to accept the new material.

THERAPEUTIC FRONTIERS

As it has in so many other serious genetic disorders, hope for more fundamental and more reliable treatments for SCID has long focused on gene therapy. But as we have seen, such "cures" have been disappointingly long in coming. Indeed, researchers have thought themselves on the verge of crossing that frontier since 1990 when the NIH gave the go-ahead for the first such attempt, and a team of physicians and medical researchers treated a four-year-old girl named Ashanti DeSilva.[4] Ashanti had a form of SCID known as ADA deficiency, and because of it she had lived a virtually cloistered life, never able to leave home yet constantly plagued with colds and other mild infections. With her

117

parents' permission, doctors at the NIH in Bethesda, Maryland, withdrew some of Ashanti's blood, separated out her mature T cells, and mixed them with a virus bearing the missing genetic instruction for producing the ADA enzyme. When a bumper crop—an estimated billion—corrected T cells had been produced in the laboratory, the doctors transfused them back into Ashanti's bloodstream.

Excitement was very high, not only in the American medical community but around the world. Dr. W. French Anderson, the lead investigator, has since remarked that "we had ourselves all hyped up, thinking there would be rapid, quick, easy, early cures." But though Ashanti has since lived a near normal life, she has never been able to cut herself free from treatments permanently. Today the circulating levels of gene-corrected T cells in Ashanti's bloodstream hover around 20 percent to 25 percent of what most people have. To maintain even this degree of immunity, the fourteen-year-old must submit to periodic reinfusions and take a variety of supportive medications. And the record until very recently has hardly been better for any other experimental subjects. Since the excitement that attended Ashanti's initial clinical trial in 1990, some four hundred other trials have been conducted worldwide, involving more than four thousand patients with various genetic disorders. Over the next ten years that passed, however, not one fulfilled Dr. Anderson's high hopes. And in a handful of examples, human gene therapy has had drastic consequences, including death.

A RISKY BUSINESS

During the summer of 1999, eighteen-year-old Jesse Gelsinger of Tucson, Arizona, volunteered to help in experiments being carried out at the University of

Pennsylvania's Institute of Human Gene Therapy. The institute was the largest academic gene therapy program in the United States, and it had a sterling reputation for the quality of its work. Jesse's case was of interest to the institute because he had ornithine transcarbamoylase deficiency (OTC), a rare metabolic disorder in which one of the five enzymes essential in ridding the body of ammonia is missing or is present in insufficient amounts.[5] Researchers at the institute believed they had developed a very promising gene therapy for OTC, but they needed consenting adults as trial subjects before they could get approval to try it on the most critical group of patients, babies.

OTC occurs in one of every 40,000 births and is typically an X-factor genetic mutation passed on by mothers to their sons. Most of the babies who inherit it die within the first year, their brain poisoned by a toxic buildup of ammonia. Jesse had been one of OTC's lucky ones. Diagnosed with the disorder early on, he was what scientists call a "mosaic," meaning that while the majority of his cells lacked the critical enzyme, enough cells did produce ornithine transcarbamoylase naturally to keep him asymptomatic if he kept to a low-protein diet and took his medications. Thus, Jesse would not stand to benefit particularly from what doctors learned, though he certainly liked the idea that he might be able to get off his restrictive diet if the treatment worked. As a caring young man, what drew him to participate was the idea that he could contribute to the development of a new drug that would help future infants diagnosed with OTC to live and perhaps to be healthy. He and the seventeen other participants in the study had been led to believe that the experiment posed no threat to health other than contracting a transient case of flu and perhaps some mild inflammation of the liver, both of which would rapidly cure themselves. A multitude of animal studies that had preceded the human trials seemed to be evidence that this assertion was true enough.

Consequently, the teenager was relaxed when he showed up at the hospital for a battery of preliminary tests. And he was cheerful when on September 13, virtually ten years from the day Ashanti had begun her gene therapy, the geneticists carried out the experiment. Jesse was strapped to a table, sedated, and then two slim catheters were inserted in his groin. Over the next two hours, 30 milliliters of prepared genetic "soup" were pumped into his body. The soup consisted of weakened cold viruses, which were the vectors, with corrective genes for manufacturing the ornithine transcarbamoylase enzyme embedded within them.

The night following the procedure, Jesse Gelsinger spiked a high fever and felt general discomfort, but the symptoms all fell within the description of temporary reactions, and neither the doctors nor Jesse was particularly concerned. But by the next morning, however, Jesse was mentally confused, as though something more serious was going on. (Remember that one of the chief ways that OTC expresses itself is as a buildup of toxic ammonia in the brain.) By afternoon, Jesse had fallen into a coma, and over the next several days, he slid into multiple organ system failure. A test on Friday, September 17, showed that Jesse was brain dead. His incredulous parents asked that life support be removed to let him die in peace.

Jesse's death shocked the entire research community and triggered a host of investigations by the NIH and the FDA. They prudently put all further activities in gene therapy on hold, not only at the Pennsylvania Institute but everywhere else, until answers could be found. During a series of hearings, they looked at practices at every laboratory under their control. The review board found that too many of these efforts were forging ahead recklessly and that spokesmen were making inflated claims about their successes in an effort apparently to maintain financial support of the studies and attract participants. The reviewers further discovered that the kind of scientific oversight that normally requires investigators to prove clinical benefit before proceeding was not observed with any consistency. Though regulations were quite specific regarding the need to report adverse events associated with gene therapy trials, such rules were not uniformly followed. More specifically, the board found that Jesse Gelsinger's multiple organ system failure was not the first time that patients involved in the University of Pennsylvania studies had experienced serious side effects, none of which had been accurately reported. Mental confusion, mild strokes, and alterations in blood chemistry were just some of the other events that had rolled out of gene therapy experiments, which had not yielded any measurable improvements in patients' disorders. Similarly disturbing facts were uncovered at other research centers. Despite paying lip service to the Hippocratic oath "to do no harm," harm had indeed been done many times. As one of the investigators on the NIH panel remarked with notable understatement, "Gene therapy is not yet *therapy*."

Two years later, gene therapy seems to be back on track, but with less hype, more regulation, and better science guiding it. Recent work at France's Hôpital Necker-Enfants Malades gives all of us good reason for renewed optimism.[6]

FINALLY, SOME GOOD NEWS

In April 2000, the news about gene therapy turned positive for the first time in a decade.[7] Dr. Alain Fischer, chief of pediatric immunology at Paris's Hôpital Necker-Enfants Malades, the oldest pediatric hospital in the world, announced that he and his team had successfully corrected the immune function in two infant boys.[8] The physicians had devised a novel approach to inserting the corrective gene: instead of inserting mature T lymphocytes and B lymphocytes and hoping that they would multiply to create a healthy immune system, they had relied on undifferentiated stem cells. (Stem cells are nursery or precursor cells, capable of developing into virtually any one of the other sorts of cells the body uses, including immune cells, depending on the genetic instructions they receive.) Fischer reasoned that these precursor cells might be more amenable to manipulation.

To obtain the stem cells, Fischer took bone marrow cells from each of the babies. (Stem cells can also be harvested from the umbilical cords of newborns, and from the extra embryos that are produced in the most advanced forms of in vitro fertilization, and their use remains highly controversial at present.) Fischer then separated the undifferentiated stem cells from the rest and put them into a nutrient-rich brew designed to help them thrive and multiply. Next he added a transport virus carrying a healthy version of the gene the babies needed if they were to have an immune system. As the stem cells divided, they naturally incorporated the virus into their descendants. The "infected" cells were then put back into the twins' systems and allowed to go to work. Within fifteen days the researchers could track positive results, as large quantities of normal B lymphocytes and T lymphocytes began to circulate. Within three months the immune-healthy babies were able to go home with their parents. Two years later the boys are still healthy, and Fischer has been able to repeat his procedures several times with similar results.

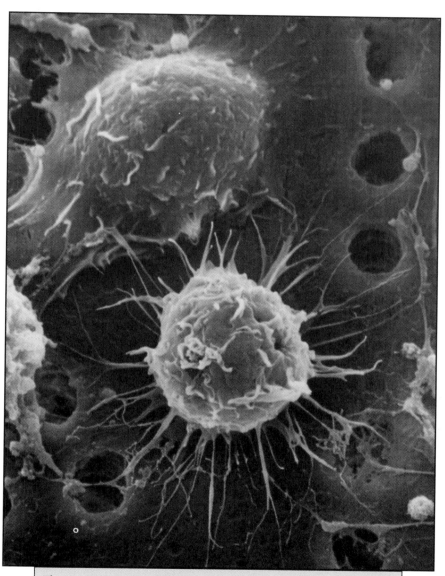

These stem cells, from human bone marrow, can travel to different parts of the body and generate bone, blood, and cartilage.

Only time will tell if the treatments produce a permanent cure or if new infusions of specially treated stem cells will have to be repeated every few years, but they have already proved far more durable than the cells given to Ashanti. Meanwhile, gene therapy researchers have been given a huge new infusion of optimism. "It does look like gene therapy might finally be turning the corner," Dr. Anderson has said in praise of his French colleagues.[9] But he went on to caution, there are still no guarantees that gene therapy will have wide application to many other disorders, rare or common. (Alzheimer's disease, Huntington's disease, Parkinson's disease, and severe spinal cord and brain damage are just a few of the other medical challenges that some researchers have mentioned as future candidates for stem cell therapy.) SCID is in Anderson's view particularly suited to the kind of genetic insertion that Fischer and his group achieved. But, he adds, "Because you correct SCID doesn't mean you can correct any other disease. On the other hand, if you can't correct SCID, you can't correct anything else, either."[10] These are indeed uncertain, exciting, and always hopeful times.

GLOSSARY

allele—genes that govern different forms of the same trait are called alleles. Since genes occur in pairs, one provided by the mother's genome and one by the father's genome, a key element in determining the expression of many disorders is whether the offspring receives two identical alleles for a particular mutation (homozygous) or two differing alleles (heterozygous).

amino acids—the building blocks of proteins.

amniocentesis—a medical procedure in which a sample of the fluid surrounding a fetus is drawn off through a hollow needle inserted in the mother's abdomen to obtain fetal cells for genetic testing. The procedure is generally done shortly after the first fifteen weeks of pregnancy.

base—one of the four molecules that form the rungs of the DNA ladder and make up the genetic code. The molecules are adenine (A), cytosine (C), guanine (G), and thymine (T).

biologics—commercial products, including drugs, derived from biotechnology.

carrier—any person who possesses one recessive gene in a gene pair. It usually refers to those having a gene for a genetic disorder.

chromosome—one of the threadlike strings of genes and other DNA found in the nucleus of a cell. Humans have twenty-three pairs of chromosomes, forty-six chromosomes in all. Of these, twenty-two pairs are "autosomes," meaning they code for the body, and one pair are sex chromosomes, meaning they are involved in determining the sex. Each parent contributes one chromosome to each pair, so a child gets half from the mother and half from the father.

cluster—a term used to identify a disease pattern among segments of the population that is statistically greater than normal.

connective tissue—tissue that supports and joins other body tissues and parts. Bone, cartilage, muscles, and tendons are all connective tissue.

deletion—the kind of mutation in which one or more bases is dropped from the DNA of a gene, typically leading to an "error."

DNA—deoxyribonucleic acid, the molecule that makes up the gene.

dominant—when the alleles for a particular trait are heterozygous, meaning they differ in some way, one of the alleles may express itself, that is, may be dominant, and mask the presence of the other allele, which is then termed recessive.

enzymes—proteins that speed up chemical reactions in cells.

fetus—a human embryo after the third month of pregnancy.

FDA—Food and Drug Administration; the federal agency responsible for overseeing the development and manufacture of drugs and medical devices as well as the management of clinical testing.

gene—the basic unit of heredity, a discrete piece of DNA.

gene therapy—an evolving group of extremely advanced procedures used to treat inherited disorders at the molecular level. The medical procedure involves either replacing, manipulating, or supplementing abnormal genes with healthy genes.

genetic code—the instructions in a gene that tell the cell how to make a specific protein. Each gene's code combines the four chemicals adenine, cytosine, guanine, and thymine in various ways to spell out the "words" that specify which amino acid is needed at every step in the making of a protein.

genetic counseling—a short-term counseling process available to individuals and families who have a genetic disease or who believe they are at risk for such a disease. Genetic counseling provides information about the subjects' condition and helps them make informed decisions.

genetic research—a two-step process in which the gene responsible for a particular abnormality is located and then deciphered in the effort to discover how it works to produce the disorder's symptoms.

genetic screening—testing a population group to identify a subset of individuals at high risk for having or transmitting a specific genetic disorder.

genetics—the study of inheritance patterns.

genome—described by Dr. Francis Collins, one of the mappers, as "the book of life," the genome contains among the welter of repetitive and meaningless DNA sequences the codes for some 30,000 working genes that are the essential controls of human life.

insertion—the kind of mutation in which one or more bases is added to the DNA of a gene.

linkage—genes that, in lying close together on the same chromosome, often are passed on together.

Mendelian inheritance—the manner in which genes and traits are passed from parents to offspring. Named for Gregor Mendel, a nineteenth-century pioneer in plant studies.

multifactorial—a characteristic determined by a combination of genes and environment.

mutation—a change in a gene that alters its function in any way. Mutations may be caused by random assortment, by chemical intervention, by radiation, by a virus, or by some other environmental variable. Mutations may take the form of a deletion, an insertion, or a substitution. If a particular mutation codes for a protein essential to life, it may cause the fetus to die in the womb or shortly after birth; if, as is the case more often, it codes for a somewhat less essential protein or hormone, it may not cause early death but its effects can be serious nonetheless, showing up as one of the many orphan diseases.

NORD—National Organization for Rare Disorders, an alliance of voluntary health organizations and individuals dedicated to helping people with rare disorders.

population—in genetics, a term denoting the size of a group being studied for the statistical frequency of a particular disorder.

prognosis—a medical assessment of the probable course and outcome of a disease. It is based on a number of factors, including the recorded history of others with the same disease and the individual's general condition and age.

rare disorder—defined by the FDA as a disorder or disease shared by no more than 200,000 Americans. In some cases, there may be as few as a thousand or even a hundred people so afflicted.

recessive—a gene that is masked by a dominant gene or allele. A recessive gene will show its effects when it is paired with a similar recessive gene (i.e., both mother's and father's) in the offspring. The term is also used to describe the pattern of inheritance associated with a recessive gene.

sex-linked—a gene carried on the X chromosome, or the pattern of inheritance associated with a gene carried on the X chromosome. Sex-linked (or X-linked) disorders are generally expressed only in males though females are frequently carriers.

spectrum—when the degree of disability within a particular disorder varies greatly from mild to severe, the range is referred to as a spectrum.

syndrome—when a disorder has multiple symptoms occurring together, it is often referred to as a syndrome.

substitution—a mutation in which one base is inserted in place of another in the DNA of a gene.

tic—a brief, repetitive, purposeless, involuntary movement or sound. Motor tics are tics that produce twitches; tics that produce sounds are called phonic tics. Tics may also be simple or complex, depending on whether they involve one tic or multiple variations. Coprolalia is a complex phonic tic in which the individual compulsively blurts out offensive and socially inappropriate phrases; though often associated with Tourette syndrome, it is in fact a rare manifestation of that disorder.

CHAPTER NOTES

Introduction
William Harvey, *The Works of William Harvey* (London: 1847 edition), p. 616.

Chapter One
1. Sheryl Gay Stolberg, "In 'Mother Teresa's Waiting Room,' Optimism," *New York Times*, April 14, 1999, p. A18.

2. Speech by Abbey S. Meyers, president of NORD, at the International Conference of Rare Diseases and Orphan Drugs, February 18, 2000.

3. John Henkel, "Orphan Drug Law Matures into Mainstay," *FDA Consumer*, Vol. 33, No. 3 (May-June 1999), pp. 29–33.

4. NORD database, www.rarediseases.org

Chapter Two

1. Jasmine Lee O'Neill, special article prepared for the National Autistic Society Web site at http://www.oneworld.org/autism_uk/peoplew/jasmine.html

2. Uta Frith, *Autism, Explaining the Enigma*, Oxford, UK: Blackwell, 1992, p. 32ff.

3. "An Unlikely Virtuoso: Leslie Lemke and the Story of the Savant Syndrome," *The Sciences* (January/February 1988), pp. 28–35.

4. "Genius Among Us: Profile of Alonzo Clemons," at www.wismed.org/foundation/clemons.htm

5. Personal communication with Ruth C. Sullivan, Joseph's mother and founder of Autism Services Center, Huntington, West Virginia.

6. Darrold Treffert, MD, "Rain Man, the Movie/Rain Man, Real Life" posted at www.wismed.org/foundation/rainman.htm

7. Temple Grandin, "Thinking in Pictures: Autism and Visual Thought," posted at www.grandin.com/inc/visual.thinking.html, p. 1.

8. Wendy Lawson, "Don't Take It Literally," special article prepared for the National Autistic Society Web site at www.oneworld.org/autism_uk/peoplew/wendy.html

9. Temple Grandin, "An Inside View of Autism," at www.autism.org/temple/inside.html, p. 2.

10. Sandra Blakeslee, "Movement May Offer Early Clue to Autism," *New York Times*, January 26, 1999, p. F3.

11. Sandra Blakeslee, "4 Brain Chemicals . . . ," *New York Times*, May 4, 2000, p. F2.

12. Maria Newman, "No Environmental Causes Found . . . ," *New York Times*, April 19, 2000, p. B4.

13. Dean E. Murphy, "Crimes of Passion . . . ," *New York Times*, March 15, 2001, p. B6.

14. "*Struggling With Life*," a summary of an ABC News story broadcast on *Prime Time*, October 26, 2000.

15. Murphy, p. B6.

Chapter Four

1. Randi Henderson and Marjorie Centofanti, "Life as a Little Person," *Hopkins Medical News* (Spring-Summer 1995), p. 1.

2. Little People of America, "*Position Statement on Genetic Discoveries in Dwarfism*," posted at Web site: psy-138-006.bsd.uchicago.edu

3. Gillian Mueller, "Extended Limb-Lengthening/ Setting the Record Straight" article posted at www2.shore.net/—dkennedy//dwarfism_gillian.html (July 3, 2000).

Chapter Five

1. Cystic Fibrosis Foundation, "Special People 2001: Darrell Hedgecoth Triumphs Despite Triple Transplant," posted at www.cff.org/special people01.htm

2. Amy Bland, Kevin Gibson, Angela Mayorga et al., "Cystic Fibrosis," a paper posted at medicine.creighton.edu/forpatients/CF/cf.html

3. "Facts About Cystic Fibrosis," posted at www.cff.org/facts.htm

4. *New York Times*, Obituaries, "John O'Brien," May 2, 2001, p. C15.

5. "Genetic Screening for Tay-Sachs Disease," posted at www.seas.upenn.edu:8080/~rogerwal/roger3.html

6. *New York Times*, Obituaries, "John O'Brien," p. C15.

Chapter Six

1. T.J. Murray quoting Boswell in "Medical History of Dr. Samuel Johnson's...disorder," *British Medical Journal*, 1974, pp. 1610–1614.
2. Ibid.
3. Erica Goode, "Most Ills Are a Matter of More Than One Gene," *New York Times*, June 27, 2000, p. F1.
4. John Cade biography posted at Web site: www.vh.org
5. Michael J. Aminoff, *Electrodiagnosis in Clinical Neurology*, 2 ed. (New York: Churchill Livingston, 1986), pp. 6–7.

Chapter Seven

1. Steve McVicker, "Bursting the Bubble," posted on Houston Press Online, posted April 10, 1997 at www.houstonpress.com/issues/1997-04-10/features.html
2. "Overview of Primary Immune Deficiency Diseases," as posted at www.primaryimmune.org/b02.htm
3. Immune Deficiency Foundation homepage posted at www.scid.net
4. Larry Thompson, "Human Gene Therapy," *FDA Consumer*, Vol. 34, No. 5 (September–October 2000), p. 19.
5. *New York Times Sunday Magazine*, November 28, 1999, "The Biotech Death of Jesse Gelsinger," by Sheryl Gay Stolberg, posted at www.gene.ch/gen-tech/1999/Dec/msg00005.html

6. Homepage, Hôpital Necker-Enfants Malades, found at www.ap-hop-paris.fr

7. Gina Kolata, "In a First, Gene Therapy Saves Lives of Infants," *The New York Times* on the Web, April 28, 2000. http://www.nytimes.com

8. Thompson, p. 24.

9. Kolata, *The New York Times* on the Web, April 28, 2000.

10. Kolata.

FOR FURTHER READING

Aminoff, Michael J., MD. *Electrodiagnosis in Clinical Neurology*, 2nd ed. New York: Churchill Livingstone, 1986.

Basara, Lisa Ruby, RPh, and Michael Montagne, RPh. *Searching for Magic Bullets: Consumer Activism and Pharmaceutical Development.* New York: Haworth Press, 1995.

Bunch, Bryan, ed. *The Family Encyclopedia of Disease.* New York: W.H. Freeman and Company, 1998.

Byrd, W. Michael, and Linda A. Clayton. *An American Health Dilemma, A Medical History of African Americans and The Problem of Race.* New York: Routledge, 2000.

Frith, Uta. *Autism, Explaining the Enigma.* Oxford, UK: Blackwell, 1992.

Grandin, Temple. *Emergence: Labeled Autistic*. New York: Warner Books, 1996.

————*Thinking in Pictures and Other Reports from My Life with Autism*. New York: Vintage Books, 1996.

Harre, Rom, and Roger Lamb, eds. *The Dictionary of Physiological and Clinical Psychology*. Cambridge, MA: The MIT Press, 1986.

Mulvihill, Mary Lou, PhD. *Human Diseases*, 2nd ed. Norwalk, CT: Appleton & Lange, 1987.

Murphy, Wendy et al., eds. *The Brain*. Alexandria, VA: Time-Life Books and St. Remy Press, 1990.

National Organization for Rare Disorders (NORD). *Rare Disorders Database*. New Fairfield, CT.

"Orphan Disease Update," NORD newsletters, Vol. 12-19, 1995–2001, New Fairfield, CT.

Park, Clara Claiborne. *The Siege*. New York: Harcourt Brace & World, 1968.

Rapoport, Judith L., MD. *The Boy Who Couldn't Stop Washing, The Experience and Treatment of Obsessive-Compulsive Disorder*. New York: E.P. Dutton, 1989.

Steadman's Medical Dictionary, 26th ed. Baltimore, MD: Williams & Wilkins, 1995.

Zallen, Doris Teichler. *Does It Run in the Family, Consumer's Guide to DNA Testing for Genetic Disorders*. New Brunswick, NJ: Rutgers University Press, 1997.

INTERNET RESOURCES

Virtually every medical disorder is served by one or more Web sites. Many of these sites focus on a single condition to the exclusion of others and include a number of services of unique value to individuals with the rare diseases as well as their families and medical support teams. The Cystic Fibrosis Foundation (www.cff.org), the Little People of America (www.lpaonline.org), and the Osteogenesis Imperfecta Foundation (www.oif.org) are excellent examples. Other Web sites where good information may be found are certain pharmaceutical research companies and hospitals where specific work in some rare disorders is ongoing. Below is a list of highly reliable but more broadly focused resources where you may begin your searches:

Centers for Disease Control and Prevention:
www.cdc.gov

138

Children of Difference: www.childrenofdifference.org

Food and Drug Administration (FDA): www.fda.gov

Hereditary Disease Foundation, Inc.: www.hdfoundation.org

Little People of America: www.lpaonline.org

March of Dimes Birth Defects Foundation: www.modimes.org

National Center for Biotechnology Information: www.ncbi.nlm.nih.gov

National Heart, Lung and Blood Institute: www.nhlbi.nih.gov

National Human Genome Research Institute: www.nhgri.nih.gov

National Institute of Arthritis and Musculoskeletal and Skin Diseases: www.niams.nih.gov

National Institute of Child Health and Human Development: www.nichd.nih.gov

National Institute on Deafness and Other Communication Disorders: www.nidcd.nih.gov

National Institute of Diabetes and Digestive and Kidney Diseases: www.niddk.nih.gov

National Institute of Neurological Disorders and Stroke: www.ninds.nih.gov

National Organization for Rare Disorders, Inc.: www.rarediseases.org

Office of Orphan Products Development: www.fda.gov/orphan/

WebMD-Health: my.webmd.com

INDEX

Page numbers in *italics* refer to illustrations.

AZT, 19

Bester, Madge, 78
Bipolar disorder (manic depression), 99, 102–108
Bisphosphates, 80
Bone-marrow transplantation, 60–61, 117
Boswell, James, 95
Break bone disorder (*see* Osteogenesis imperfecta)
Buckley, Rebecca, 116–117
Bulimia, 99

Cade, John, 106
Centers for Disease Control and Prevention (CDC), 30, 47
Chromosomes, 23
Clemons, Alonzo, 35
Clomipramine (Anafranil), 101
Cold viruses, 88
Collagen, 77
Collins, Francis S., 87
Computational biology, 25
Cri du Chat syndrome, 21
Cystic fibrosis (CF), 81–89
    diagnosis of, 84
    gene responsible for, 25, 87
    incidence of, 81, 82
    treatment of, *83*, 84–88
Cystic Fibrosis Foundation, 85, 88–89
Cystic fibrosis transmembrane conductance regulator (CFTR), 87, 88
Cytosine, 23

Deficiency anemias, 64–65
DeSilva, Ashanti, 117–118, 120, 124
Desire for sameness, 32, 33–34
DNA (deoxyribonucleic acid), 22–23, 57
Dominant gene, 24, 26
Dopamine, 105
Down, J. Langdon, 34–35
Drugs (*see* Medications)
Dwarfism (*see* Achondroplasia)

Ekstein, Josef, 92–93
Electroconvulsive therapy (ECT), 106–108, *107*
Electrophoresis, 56
Emmel, V.E., 54
Environmental factors, 24, 47
Enzymes, 23
Epidermolysis bullosa, 19
Erythropoetin, 19
Eugenics, 58–59
Exposure and response prevention, 101–102

Fanconi's anemia, 64
Fischer, Alain, 122, 124
Folic acid anemia, 64–65
Food and Drug Administration (FDA), 16, 17, 21, 60, 85, 121
    Office of Orphan Products Development, 18
    Orphan Drug Grant Program, 18
Fosamax, 80
Fuller, Thomas, 34, 35

Gelsinger, Jesse, 119–121
Gene-based medicine, 26–28
Genentech, 85
Genes, 22–26
Gene therapy, 12, 61, 117–122, 124
Genetic testing, 57–58
Genome, 12, 23
Grandin, Temple, 38–41, *42*, 46
Growth hormones, 74
Guanine, 23

Harvey, William, 9
Hassidim, 92–93
Hedgecoth, Darrell, 86
Hemoglobin, 50, 54
Hemolytic anemias, 65
Hemophilia, 10, 61, 63
Herbert, Mikki, 48
Heritable anemias, 64
Hermaphrodism, 21
Herrick, James B., 54

142